BEFORE YOU GET PREGNANT

How to Sow the Best Seeds for
Your Baby's Developing Brain

CHONG CHEN, PH.D.

Brain & Life Publishing

London

ISBN 978-1-912533-00-8 Paperback

Brain & Life Publishing

27 Old Gloucester Street, London, U.K.

First Printing, 2017

For information about special needs for bulk purchases, sales promotions, and educational needs, please contact orders@brainandlife.net.

ALSO BY CHONG CHEN

*Plato's Insight: How Physical Exercise Boosts
Mental Excellence*

*Fitness Powered Brains: Optimize Your Productivity,
Leadership and Performance*

*Psychology for Pregnancy: How Your Mental Health
during Pregnancy Programs Your Baby's Developing Brain
(Your Baby's Developing Brain Series I)*

*The Seed of Intelligence: Boost Your Baby's Developing
Brain through Optimal Nutrition and Healthy Lifestyle
(Your Baby's Developing Brain Series II)*

*The Wonder of Prenatal Education: Why You Should
Listen to Mozart and Sing to Your Baby While Pregnant
(Your Baby's Developing Brain Series III)*

To my parents for their love and support

Table of Contents

PREFACE

Given my training in medicine, psychiatry, and brain science, my family and friends have long been asking me what science says about pregnancy and parenting. For instance, how does one boost a baby's brain development? How can one raise a genius? Is there anything parents can do during pregnancy to ensure a healthy, intelligent, and happy child? To answer their questions, I did extensive research myself and after over six years, I have finally completed a series, "*Your Baby's Developing Brain*," describing what parents can do during pregnancy to protect and boost their baby's developing brain.

However, in that series I was unable to present some significant results. That is because starting to prepare for a baby's developing brain after realizing one gets pregnant is already too late. On one hand, you need an optimal physical and mental status to prepare your sperm/eggs, to make them healthy enough to be the origin of your baby's life. On the other hand, your baby needs an optimal nutritional environment the most in his first few weeks of age, when his body and brain are undergoing the fastest development. A nutritious diet and healthy body leading up to conception are critical for the optimal development of your baby.

Unfortunately, almost half of the pregnancies are actually unplanned, which puts the fetuses to substantial risks; furthermore, whereas pregnant women are generally more aware of their nutrition, most women who are trying to conceive do not have more nutritional awareness than those who are not trying to conceive, and more than half of them do not seek advice about preconception health from a healthcare professional. This serious reality drives me to write this volume, through which I want to inform women who are trying to conceive what they can do prior to pregnancy. If you are already pregnant at this moment, I would also recommend you read this book in order for you to realize the potential risk you may have subjected your baby to and the seriousness of achieving a health revolution immediately.

CHAPTER 1
Plan Your Pregnancy at Least Three Months Ahead

To prepare for your baby's developing brain, parents should start preparing yourselves at least three months ahead. Parents with medical conditions in particular may have to prepare longer, for instance, half a year to more than one year. Here are the reasons:

Fathers, prepare your sperm

Research in the past 15 years has been telling us that a man's life experiences, such as health and lifestyle, leave imprints in his sperm. A man with a healthy body weight and lifestyle including a nutritious diet and no negative habits such as smoking or alcohol drinking, tends to have more and healthier sperm, which, after fertilization, eventually grows into a healthy child. As new sperm are made every 42–76 days, damaged sperm can be replaced within three months of a "health revolution." A minimum of three months for preconception health revolution offers a window of opportunity for the future fathers to optimize their sperm. Below is a more detailed account of the evidence.

Sperm DNA can be damaged by an unhealthy lifestyle, medical conditions, and exposure to environmental risks, as listed below. They reduce sperm count and quality.

- *Poor diet*: low-protein diet, high saturated fat diet, folate deficiency, zinc deficiency, high caffeine intake, smoking, and heavy alcohol drinking, among other things

- *Medical conditions*: obesity, untreated diabetes mellitus, sleep problems, chronic inflammation for instance caused by infections, psychological issues including stress, depression, and anxiety

- *Drugs and exposures*: anabolic steroids, antibiotics, marijuana, cocaine, radiation, chemotherapy, metals (e.g., lead, cadmium), organic solvents (e.g., glues, paints), and many xenobiotics including acrylamide (produced during frying, baking, and overcooking) and polychlorinated bi-phenyls (PCBs)

Such damage results in infertility or subfertility (not achieving pregnancy in six months). However, pregnancy may still be possible despite some DNA damage and can result in spontaneous abortions, birth defects, and many other diseases including childhood cancers. Here, another mechanism—epigenetics—works.

Epigenetics refers to a collection of processes that control gene expression without changing nucleotide sequence. DNA methylation is one such process by which methyl groups are added to the DNA molecule and when located in a gene promoter, DNA methylation typically represses gene transcription. DNA methylation is essential for normal development and functioning, but abnormal DNA methylation is associated with many diseases including cancer, asthma, metabolic and various mental disorders. Recently, it has been realized that germ line epigenetic modifications can be inherited from parents to offspring and is responsible for the intergenerational transmission of diseases.

For instance, as discovered by public health specialist Adelheid Soubry at Duke University, paternal obesity at the time of conception is linked with hypomethylation at the differentially methylated regions (DMR) of the insulin-like growth factor 2 (IGF2) gene in their newborn offspring. When the IGF2 DMR is hypomethylated, there is increased circulation of IGF2 proteins, which are associated with increased likelihood of obesity. In other words, through such epigenetic mechanism, parternal obesity at the time of conception increases the risk of offspring obesity. Meanwhile, paternal overweight at the time of conception has been associated with higher breast cancer risk in daughters, while a parental diet high in saturated fats before conception is associated with a higher risk of obesity and diabetes in the offspring.

By the same tone, even in the absence of maternal drinking, paternal heavy alcohol drinking shortly before conception induces germ line epigenetic changes that cause physiologic and behavioral abnormalities in offspring. One such epigenetic change is the reduced expression of a key enzyme catalyzing DNA methylation called DNA methyltransferase 1. The results of such epigenetic changes range from increased perinatal mortality, low birth weight and length, increased malformations, decreased spatiotemporal learning ability, and higher levels of depressive symptoms.

Therefore, as a father-to-be, plan beforehand; remove all your risks and achieve a health revolution. This will dramatically increase your chances of having a healthy baby.

Mothers, prepare your eggs and body

Similarly, a woman's health and lifestyle affect her eggs and determine her health status. Eggs do not renew themselves in mammals. Females have a fixed amount of primordial follicles or oocytes (which are immature egg cells) at birth (1–2 million in humans). That is, a woman's oocytes are formed only during her own fetal life. At reproductive age, the maturation of oocytes takes an estimated 85 days in humans and on average one oocyte completes growth each month and is released by the ovary. The released mature egg enters the fallopian tube to get fertilized by a sperm. Oocytes are affected by changes in the levels of circulating metabolites and metabolic hormones that are responsive to nutritional status and health conditions. A minimum of three months of health revolution prior to conception provides an opportunity for the mother to renew and optimize her eggs.

Besides changing the unhealthy lifestyles listed above, a well-balanced nutritious diet (see Chapter 2) is recommended as it promotes oocytes maturity and improves oocyte quality.

Equally important, the mother's body is the fetus's growth environment, so the mother's health and nutrition before and during pregnancy is her baby's health and nutrition. Most notably, it has been a routine practice worldwide that in order to prevent neural tube defect and promote fetal health, pregnant women take folate acid and iron supplement starting two months before the planned pregnancy and throughout the duration of the pregnancy.

Folic acid is a B vitamin that plays an important role in DNA synthesis. It is particularly important for the development of the fetal spine, brain, and skull during the first four weeks of pregnancy. Low folic acid levels around the time of conception may cause neural tube defects in infants. Neural tube defects involve the failure of the neural tube—the precursor of fetal spine and brain—to close properly. Neural tube defects typically occur during the third and fourth week of pregnancy, before the woman knows she is pregnant. Research shows that this risk is substantially reduced when the mother takes daily folic acid supplement prior to and throughout pregnancy.

Iron, an essential micronutrient, is necessary not only in synthesizing hemoglobin for carrying oxygen but also for forming enzymes that catalyze many processes including the biosynthesis of hormones, synapses, neurotransmission, and DNA and RNA base repair. Iron requirements during pregnancy increase substantially due to increased requirements by the placenta and the fetus. Unfortunately, about 42% of pregnant women around the world, that is, almost one in two pregnant women, are anemic. Even in well-resourced areas such as North America and Europe, the prevalence of anemia is as high as 25%, or one in four pregnant women. You can take a blood test to see if you are anemic. A blood hemoglobin level lower than 110 g/L is considered anemic. Half of the anemia is simply due to iron deficiency.

In the face of these findings, currently WHO recommends:

- Daily supplementation of 30 to 60 mg of iron plus 400 µg folic acid starting from 2 months before the planned pregnancy and throughout pregnancy for all pregnant women to prevent neural tube defects and anemia, and promote maternal and fetal health.

- For those with anemia, daily supplementation of 120 mg of iron until their blood hemoglobin levels rise to normal (after which they can resume the standard daily 30 to 60 mg of iron).

Supplementation can be fulfilled in the form of fortified foods (foods to which extra nutrients have been added) and/or supplements. This recommendation has been a standard practice around the world.

Check your health conditions

We now know that many medical conditions especially those in the mother (such as obesity, diabetes mellitus, epilepsy, asthma, hypertension, and hypothyroidism) negatively affect pregnancy and the baby's development. These medical conditions often lead to preterm birth, low birth weight, intrauterine growth restriction, and many birth defects.

Preterm birth (birth before 37 weeks gestation), low birth weight (birth weight less than 2,500 grams), and intrauterine growth restriction (poor growth of a fetus while in the womb) are often related. Infants with any one of these conditions carry a high risk of delayed physical and mental development. They are more likely to die, get various infections, be shorter at adulthood, have lower cognitive ability, achieve less at school, have lower income, and develop diabetes, cancers, and mental health problems.

In many cases, medical conditions themselves are as detrimental as treatment during pregnancy. Take obesity for example. If the mother is obese, that is, with a BMI

$\geq$ 30, she will have a greater chance of suffering from many pregnancy complications and her baby will grow suboptimally (see Chapter 8). Nevertheless, weight loss during pregnancy is not recommended as dieting or energy restriction is as detrimental to the fetus as obesity. The safest practice is that obese women lose 5–10% of their weight prior to conception, which substantially reduces the risk on the fetus. Healthy weight loss usually takes 3–6 months (see Chapter 8).

As another example, dexamethasone, a synthetic corticosteroid drug, is broadly used to treat many inflammatory conditions including rheumatoid arthritis, asthma, croup, and multiple sclerosis. However, as shown by neuroscientist Hideo Uno at the University of Wisconsin-Madison in the 1990s, just two days of dexamethasone exposure to pregnant monkeys before delivery caused massive atrophy of hippocampal cells in the infant monkeys at birth. The hippocampus is responsible for encoding episodic memory, spatial navigation, and emotional regulation. When measured at 20 months of age, these infant monkeys exhibited a 30% reduced hippocampal volume than those born to non-exposed mothers. Reduced hippocampal volume is associated with cognitive deficits and emotional disorders. Notably, the dose of dexamethasone used in this experiment was only slightly higher than the doses used in humans.

To date, we know little about the effects of taking most medications during pregnancy. This is because pregnant women are often not included in clinical trials to determine the safety of new medications. Over 90% of drugs have little information on their risk for birth defects, not to mention healthy brain development.

Thus, if you currently have any medical conditions, be sure they are under control and being treated properly before conception. Otherwise, conception should be delayed until optimal control is achieved.

Furthermore, infectious diseases such as sexually transmitted diseases (STD) require special attention, as they not only negatively affect pregnancy and the baby's development, but also can be vertically transmitted to the baby. It is strongly recommended that couples receive comprehensive medical and STD checks before conception. Take the human immunodeficiency virus (HIV) for example. After infection, there is a window period for the antigen and antibody of HIV to show up. Depending on the HIV test used, the window period may range from 1–3 months. Reliable results are only available after this window has expired.

For infectious diseases of Hepatitis B and measles, mumps, and rubella (MMR), vaccines are highly recommended for the mother before pregnancy. There is convincing evidence that giving these immunizations before pregnancy is beneficial and that they are highly effective at preventing maternal disease and vertical transmission to the fetus. Before you get pregnant, make sure you have a blood test to see if you are immune to the disease. Most women have been vaccinated as children with the MMR vaccine, but you should confirm this with your healthcare provider. If you need to get vaccinated for rubella, because of the risk to the fetus when you receive a live virus vaccine, you should also avoid becoming pregnant until one month (in Japan, the recommendation is two months) after receiving the MMR vaccine.

Now, one should understand the importance of why parents-to-be should prepare way before your planned pregnancy.

What exactly is an unplanned pregnancy?

Unfortunately, in many countries, including the United States, approximately half of pregnancies are unplanned, that is, unintended or mistimed. An unplanned pregnancy, by definition, means that the parents-to-be have not effectively used the opportunity before pregnancy to promote their own health and prevent potential risks. It means that their unborn baby does not have the most nourishing environment at the start of his life and cannot achieve his best potential.

Are you ready to get pregnant? If so, it is time to love and nurture yourself by planning and preparing your body and mind for pregnancy.

CHAPTER 2
Know the Principle of Parenting

If you want me to summarize the principle of parenting in one sentence, it will be like this:

Make every effort to give your child an enriched environment.

Enriched means rich, nourishing, and stimulating. Environment refers to that of the physical and psychological place under which the child thrives. The best practice of parenting will be exposing your child to a nutritious diet, healthy lifestyle, a warm family atmosphere, and a stimulating learning environment.

Notably, this principle holds true even when the child is in the womb, otherwise referred to as prenatal development. The womb is the living environment of the fetus. It is how the mother's health during pregnancy plays a pivotal role in determining the fetus's development. Not only the maternal lifestyle (for example, food, and medication), but also her psychological state matters. Both change the maternal metabolism and affect the developing fetus through the placental connection. Furthermore, the fetus already possesses the ability to hear and learn by middle pregnancy, when the fetus should have started to be exposed to music, sounds, words, and stories to ensure an intellectually stimulating environment. I have written extensively in the series *"Your Baby's Developing Brain"* on these topics:

- Volume 1: *Psychology for Pregnancy: How Your Mental Health during Pregnancy Programs Your Baby's Developing Brain (2017)*

- Volume 2: *The Seed of Intelligence: Boost Your Baby's Developing Brain through Optimal Nutrition and Healthy Lifestyle (2017)*

- Volume 3: *The Wonder of Prenatal Education: Why You Should Listen to Mozart and Sing to Your Baby While Pregnant (2017)*

Below, I will summarize the most essential part discussed in these volumes that also apply before pregnancy.

The developmental trajectory of your fetus and the importance of an enriched environment

The formation of a zygote marks the beginning of the new life of your baby. It then undergoes three distinct stages:

- *The pre-embryonic stage*, or the first two weeks: a period of cell division and differentiation;

- *The embryonic period*, or from week 3 to 8: a period of the formation of tissues and organs;

- *The fetal period*, or from week 9 until birth: a period of the maturation of tissues and organs and rapid growth of the body and brain.

During gestation, your baby experiences an extremely rapid development, particularly in the brain and nervous system, which is unmatched at any other stage in life.

Neurogenesis, namely the creation of neurons, initiates on embryonic day 42 and finishes by midgestation. During this period, neurogenesis can occur at a remarkable rate of over 100,000 new cells per minute. These new cells migrate and form synapses (or synaptic connections) and communicate with each other. Synapses are the substrate of memory and other cognitive processes. During the third trimester (from week 28 to birth), it is estimated that per minute around 40,000 synapses can be formed.

The fast development of your baby renders him susceptible to various influences by you, the mother.

Your physical and psychological states before and during pregnancy until delivery determine your baby's growth environment. On one hand, accompanying the rapid development of the fetus the nutritional requirement increases. This can only be fulfilled by the mother's intake. Your nutrition is your baby's nutrition. On the other hand, you produce numerous chemicals in your body, good and bad, which are dependent on your health and lifestyle, including sleep habits, physical exercise, and work. These chemicals cross the placenta and exert powerful, long-lasting impacts on your baby.

Given an enriched, nourishing, and stimulating environment such as optimal nutrition and a healthy lifestyle, your baby will thrive. Given an impoverished, stressful, and toxic environment such as poor nutrition and an unhealthy lifestyle, your baby will struggle. Therefore, an enriched environment provides the seeds for your baby's developing brain, and determines his levels of intelligence and happiness. And your nutritional status and lifestyle before and during pregnancy shape those seeds.

The seeds of your baby's developing brain: an enriched environment neurobiologically dissected

If we dissect an enriched maternal environment from a neurobiological perspective, four pillars are at the core of its components.

The first pillar is a well-balanced nutritional supply, which provides all the necessary macronutrients and micronutrients, and satisfies the requirements of the mother and fetus. Nutrients are the building blocks of our lives especially our brains.

The second pillar is an adequate level of growth factors, including the insulin-like growth factor 1 (IGF-1) and brain-derived neurotrophic factor (BDNF). IGF-1 mediates the effects of growth hormone and promotes growth in almost every cell in the body, including the placenta. BDNF supports the production, growth, differentiation, and survival of neurons. It has been shown that the maternal blood level of BDNF corresponds with that of the fetal brain.

The third pillar is a reduced level of stress hormones, particularly cortisol. Cortisol is released to cope with threats and believed to be evolutionarily adaptive.

However, exposure to high levels of cortisol damages the brain and causes many physical and psychological problems in both the mother and unborn child.

The fourth pillar is a lower level of systemic inflammation, namely lower circulating level of pro-inflammatory cytokines. Pro-inflammatory cytokines are excreted from immune-related cells upon activation of the immune system because of infection, psychological stress or unhealthy lifestyles.

High levels of cortisol and pro-inflammatory cytokines inhibit neurogenesis (the production of new neurons), impair neurotransmission (the communication between neurons, which is the substrate of all cognitive processes), and induce cognitive deficits, sickness, and depression. Chronically high levels of maternal cortisol and pro-inflammatory cytokines are toxic to the mother and fetus. It has been associated with an increased risk of maternal hypertension, poor placental functioning, fetus growth restriction, preterm birth, and low birth weight.

These four pillars are inter-correlated, each influences the rest. For instance, a healthy diet with adequate nutrition increases blood levels of growth factors while reducing that of cortisol and pro-inflammatory cytokines. As shown throughout the rest of this book, optimal maternal nutrition and a healthy lifestyle enhance these pillars and lead to optimal physical and mental outcomes in both the mother and her fetus. These outcomes are not only beneficial during pregnancy, but also have long-lasting positive impacts for years to come.

CHAPTER 3
Eat Healthily

As the saying goes, you are what you eat. Your nutrient level determines not only your fertility but also your (the mother's) ability to maintain a healthy pregnancy. During pregnancy, what the mother eats determines what is available to the fetus. Then there comes the popular saying that during pregnancy you have to "eat for two." However, "eat for two" literally means more nutritional than quantitative: you need a more balanced nutritional intake rather than an excessive caloric intake. The increase in calories during pregnancy is actually only moderate. The U.S. Institute of Medicine (2006) estimated that:

- The first trimester (the first 12 weeks): no additional caloric intake is needed.

- The second trimester (week 13–27): additional 340 kcal/day is needed.

- The third trimester (week 28 to birth): additional 452 kcal/day is needed.

As suggested by the Minister of Health Canada (2009), the extra calories needed in the second and third trimester of pregnancy can be achieved with an additional 2 to 3 snacks or food servings each day, for instance:

- Have an extra morning snack of fruit with yogurt and an extra serving of vegetables with supper

- Have an extra glass of milk with lunch and supper

Now, let's focus on this key point: a balanced nutrition intake. The question becomes "what is the most recommended diet that provides a balanced nutritional intake?"

The answer is the Mediterranean-style diet. This diet is by far the most recommended by the scientific community. The Mediterranean-style diet refers to the traditional dietary practices of countries bordering the Mediterranean Sea, including Greece, Southern Italy, and Spain. It is characterized by:

1. High intake of plant foods: vegetables, fruits, legumes, and cereals

2. High intake of olive oil as the principal source of monounsaturated fat, but low intake of saturated fat such as butter

3. Moderate intake of fish

4. Low to moderate consumption of dairy products

5. Low consumption of meat and poultry

In the original Mediterranean-style diet, wine is consumed in low to moderate amounts. However, during pregnancy alcohol should be completely avoided (see Chapter 7). Meanwhile, in the original Mediterranean-style diet, dairy foods are consumed in only low to moderate amounts. Research nevertheless shows that a high intake of dairy foods brings many health benefits (see below).

The Mediterranean-style diet promotes the four pillars of an enriched environment. It is based on the regular intake of fruits and vegetables, lean choices of protein, omega-3 polyunsaturated fatty acids (PUFA) in the form of fatty fish, whole grains, and monounsaturated fatty acid from plant oils. It is nutritionally rich and well-balanced. The abundant omega-3 PUFA contained in fatty fish increases the levels of growth factors particularly BDNF in the maternal body, buffers psychological stress and reduces the release of cortisol. Furthermore, polyphenols contained in vegetables and fruits and omega-3 PUFA contained in fatty fish are anti-inflammatory. High adherence to the Mediterranean-style diet has been associated with reduced blood concentrations of pro-inflammatory cytokines.

Thus, strict adherence to the Mediterranean-style diet is associated with lower risk of maternal obesity, hypertension, diabetes, lower levels of psychological stress, depressive and anxious symptoms, and lower risk of preterm birth. Below I'll first show you a group of research findings on the benefits of the food patterns in the Mediterranean-style diet on the development of the fetus, after which I'll explain you how these foods are best consumed.

Fruits and vegetables

Fruits and vegetables contain abundant polyphenols, which are anti-inflammatory. They also contain many key nutrients such as folate, magnesium, vitamin C, potassium, and other health-promoting, non-essential compounds such as fiber. Furthermore, consumption of fruits and vegetables generally reduces the intake of other less nutrient-rich foods. In adults, high consumption of fruits and vegetables is associated with higher cognitive function and a lower risk of chronic diseases such as cardiovascular disease and cancer.

During pregnancy, as shown by a Canadian birth cohort study by Francois V. Bolduc at the University of Alberta, each additional daily serving of fruits (either whole fruits or 100% fruit juice) consumed by the mother was associated with a significant improvement in the cognitive development of the offspring at 1 year of age.

The U.S. Department of Agriculture and Department of Health and Human Services recommend 2 cups (3–4 servings) of fruit per day for women and men at reproductive age. 1 cup of fruit can be either 1 cup of whole fruit or 100% fruit juice (about 8 oz. or 237 ml). Whole fruit includes raw, cooked, canned, frozen, and dried. The following amounts count as 1 cup of fruit:

- 1 small apple about 6 cm in diameter

- 1 large peach of 7 cm in diameter

- 1 large orange of 7.5 cm in diameter

- 1 medium grapefruit of 10 cm in diameter

- 1 large banana about 20 cm long

- 8 large strawberries

- 14 grapes

Meanwhile, with regard to vegetables, the U.S. Department of Agriculture and Department of Health and Human Services recommend 2.5 cups (4–5 servings) per day for women and 3 cups (6–7 servings) per day for men at reproductive age. This should include vegetables of different types and colors such as dark green (broccoli, spinach, leafy salad greens), red and orange (tomatoes, carrots, pumpkins), legumes (beans and peas), and starchy (potatoes, corn, cassava). This can be taken in all forms, either raw, cooked, frozen, canned, and dried, and includes vegetable juices. For instance, the following amounts count as 1 cup of vegetables:

- 1 large green or red pepper about 8 cm in diameter

- 1 large tomato about 8 cm in diameter

- 1 large ear of corn about 20 cm long

- 2 medium carrots

- 2 large stalks of celery about 30 cm long

- 3 spears of broccoli about 13 cm long

Notably, in the case of raw leafy greens, 2 cups of raw leafy greens are considered equal to 1 cup of raw or cooked vegetables or vegetable juice.

Protein

Every cell in our body contains protein. Protein is necessary for making enzymes, hormones, and neurotransmitters. A healthy intake of protein includes a variety of protein-rich foods from both animal and plant sources, including seafood, lean meats and poultry, eggs, legumes (beans and peas), nuts, seeds, and soy products.

The recommended amount of proteins consumed per day is 5.5 ounces (about 156 grams) equivalents of protein food for women and 6.5 ounces (about 184 grams) for men. The following amounts are considered as 1 ounce-equivalent of protein food:

- 1 ounce (28 gram) of cooked meat (lean beef, pork, or ham), poultry (chicken or turkey, without skin) or fish (e.g., salmon, trout, sardines)

- 1/4 cup cooked beans

- 1/4 cup (about 2 ounces, 28 gram) of tofu

- 1 egg

- 1 tablespoon of peanut butter

- 1/2 ounce (14 gram) of nuts or seeds (e.g., 12 almonds, 24 pistachios, 7 walnut halves)

Note that protein-rich foods are rich in nutrients in addition to protein, including B vitamins, vitamin D, E, iron, omega-3 PUFA, selenium, choline, copper, zinc, and phosphorus. As seafood provides almost all of the omega-3 PUFA, to achieve a balanced diet, eat seafood regularly.

Seafood

Coldwater, fatty fish such as salmon, herring, and sardines are rich in omega-3 PUFA and vitamin D. In adults, a high intake of these fish is associated with better cognitive functions and reduced risk of cardiovascular diseases. According to the Avon Longitudinal Study of Parents and Children involving over 14,500 pregnancies in the Bristol area of U.K., high consumption of fish by the mother during pregnancy is associated with less depressive and anxious symptoms in the mother and many positive outcomes in the offspring, including:

- A lower risk of intrauterine growth restriction

- Better communication skills at 15 months

- Higher visual-spatial ability at 3 years

- Better fine motor skills (such as reaching, grasping) and social development at 3.5 years

- More altruistic behavior at 7 years

- A higher verbal IQ at 8 years

The U.S. Department of Health and Human Services recommends that men and women should consume 8–12 ounces (227–340 gram, cooked, edible portion) of a variety of seafood per week. This is about 2–3 servings a week. Importantly, seafood choices should be restricted to those lower in methylmercury.

- Preferred choices: anchovy, Atlantic croaker, Atlantic mackerel, black sea bass, butterfish, catfish, clam, cod, crab, crawfish, flounder, haddock, hake, herring, lobster (American and spiny), mullet, Pacific chub mackerel, Pacific oysters, perch (freshwater and ocean), pickerel, plaice, Pollock, salmon, sardines, scallop, skate, shad, shrimp, smelt, sole, squid, tilapia, trout (freshwater), whitefish, whiting

- Try to avoid the following because of the high likelihood of contamination by methylmercury: swordfish, shark, king mackerel, marlin, orange roughy, tuna and tilefish

Dairy

Dairy contains rich nutrients including protein, calcium, monounsaturated fatty acids, vitamin A, the B-group vitamins, vitamin D, iodine, choline, potassium, magnesium, zinc and IGF-1. Milk is the only food that contains approximately all the essential nutrients that humans need. Research has shown that high dairy intake reduces the risk of hypertension, cancer, and diabetes. During pregnancy, maternal high intake of yogurt has been associated with low levels of depressive symptoms as well.

But since dairy also contains saturated fatty acids, which are high in calories and raise blood cholesterol levels, it is recommended that choices of dairy should be fat-free or low-fat (1%).

The U.S. Department of Agriculture and Department of Health and Human Services recommend 3 cups of fat-free or low-fat dairy foods per day for all adults. These foods include milk, yogurt, milk-based desserts, cheese, and/or fortified soy beverages. Foods such as cream cheese, cream, and butter which are made from milk but have little to no calcium do not count. 1 cup of dairy food is equivalent to:

- 1 cup (8 fluid ounces or 237 ml) of milk, yogurt, or soymilk (soy beverage)

- 1 cup pudding made with milk

- 1.5 cups ice cream (1 scoop of ice cream is equivalent to 1/3 cup of milk)

- 1.5 ounces (43g) of natural cheese, or 2 ounces (57g) of processed cheese

It must be noted that sweetened dairy products (flavored milk, yogurt, drinkable yogurt, desserts) contain added sugars and may count against your daily calorie limits (for daily calorie needs, see Chapter 8).

Abandon "Western" diets

The Western diet is characterized by high consumption of red, processed meats (e.g., sausages, luncheon meats, bacon, and beef jerky, which are products preserved by smoking, curing, salting, and the addition of chemical preservatives), fast foods (high saturated fat and salt), refined grains, sweets, soft drinks, and salty snacks. That is, it is full of high saturated fats, sugar, and salt.

In the general population, high consumption of red, processed meat has been associated with increased risk of cardiovascular diseases, cancer, and diabetes. High intake of fast foods, sweets, soft drinks, and salty snacks has been associated with obesity.

During pregnancy, a maternal western diet has been associated with:

- A higher risk of gestational diabetes mellitus

- Higher levels of maternal stress and depressive symptom both during and after pregnancy

- Higher risk of a small for gestational-age infant (indicating restricted fetal growth)

- More aggressive behaviors and symptoms of attention deficit hyperactivity disorder (ADHD) at 1.5 and 3 years of age in the offspring

Furthermore, maternal high intake of sweets and soft drinks is associated with excessive weight gain during pregnancy and increased risk of obesity in their offspring.

To read more about a healthy diet, get a copy of *Dietary Guidelines for Americans 2015-2020* (Eighth edition, https://health.gov/dietaryguidelines/2015/guidelines) and another book I wrote for pregnant women *The Seed of Intelligence: Boost Your Baby's Developing Brain through Optimal Nutrition and Healthy Lifestyle.*

CHAPTER 4
Be Physically Active

As demonstrated by modern medicine, psychology, and neuroscience, regular physical exercise perhaps is the most powerful strategy towards optimal health and a productive brain.

Physical exercise enhances cognitive functions and boosts work performance

Vegetables, fruits, and a better living environment are expensive. Taking this into consideration, improving work performance is highly important. How then can one boost work performance? The answer is by making one's brain more efficient. Engaging in regular physical exercise provides a solution.

At the neural level, regular exercise increases the efficiency of the prefrontal cortex, which is the CEO of our brain and is critical for reasoning and problem-solving. It also increases the number of newborn neurons in the hippocampus, an area of the brain responsible for episodic memory and spatiotemporal skills.

In an experiment conducted by David Frew at Gannon University and Nealia Bruning at Kent State University, commercial real estate stock brokers who attended a 12-week exercise program had higher sales during and after the program as opposed to their colleagues who did not attend. The 12-week program consisted of merely walking and running thrice weekly. In another observational study conducted by Jim McKenna at Leeds Metropolitan University in the U.K., on days when the workers exercised, their time management skills, mental performance and ability to meet deadlines increased. Overall, the study showed that exercise led to a boost in job performance by approximately 15%.

Regular exercise boosts the efficiency of the brain and improves work performance. If you want to read more about this topic, refer to *Fitness Powered Brains: Optimize Your Productivity, Leadership and Performance (2017).*

Maternal exercise promotes fetal development

There are more benefits of regular exercise on pregnancy. Firstly, regular exercise possesses therapeutic effects to many medical conditions that compromise fertility, such as stress, obesity, and diabetes mellitus.

Secondly, during pregnancy, exercise benefits both the mother and fetus. To the mother, regular exercise prevents excessive weight gain and many pregnancy complications including preeclampsia (a condition characterized by high blood pressure and damage to another organ system such as the liver and kidneys) and gestational diabetes, and reduces her levels of stress and negative emotions (see Chapter 11).

Thirdly, regular exercise powerfully reduces systemic inflammation, buffers physiological response to stress, and increases the levels of growth factors. Therefore, regular exercise sows the seeds for your baby's developing brain. It has been reported that infants born to mothers who engaged in physical exercise for 2.5 hours per week—or 30 minutes a day for five days a week—during pregnancy:

- Are more likely to show high vocabulary ability at 15 months of age.

- Possess overall higher language ability at 2 years of age.

Aerobic or resistance exercise?

Physical exercise is beneficial. Then what kind of exercise should you do, aerobic or resistance? Aerobic exercise, also known as endurance activity or cardiovascular exercise, involves a sustained period of rhythmic movement of large muscles. It requires the pumping of oxygenated blood by the heart to deliver oxygen to the muscles to generate energy. Examples of aerobic exercise include walking, jogging, running, cycling, swimming, dancing, playing soccer, basketball, tennis, and more. Resistance exercise, or anaerobic exercise, is brief muscle-strengthening activities, such as sprinting, jumping, weightlifting, pushups, and sit-ups. It involves major muscle groups of the legs, hips, back, abdomen, chest, shoulders, and arms.

Regarding benefits on cognitive functions and memory, research suggests aerobic exercise is better than resistance exercise. In contrast, regarding benefits on relieving stress and enhancing mood, resistance exercise is better than aerobic exercise. Moreover, several recent studies suggest that aerobic and resistance exercise may have different influences on growth factors. Whereas aerobic exercise increases serum levels of BDNF, resistance exercise increases serum level of IGF-1. Thus, aerobic and resistance exercise may benefit you and your fetus through different molecular mechanisms. Combined training of aerobic and resistance exercise will have the largest impact on you and your unborn child. So rather than worry about which kind of exercise brings the biggest benefits, do both.

The recommended amount of exercise

Currently, various international and national guidelines recommend adults to do at least 150 minutes of moderate-intensity or 75 minutes of vigorous-intensity aerobic exercise, or an equivalent combination of both weekly. Moderate-intensity aerobic exercise may include brisk walking, double tennis, table tennis, gardening, or ballroom dancing. Vigorous-intensity aerobic exercise may include jogging, single tennis, or swimming. With regard to resistance exercise, at least 20 minutes of resistance exercise three times a week, such as sprinting, weightlifting, pushups, sit-ups, and jumping is recommended.

Nevertheless, for pregnant women, activities that may lead to abdominal injury or falling, such as weightlifting, horse riding, judo, skiing or skating should be avoided. Read more about several national guidelines on physical exercise at https://brainandlife.net/exercise.

CHAPTER 5
Sleep Soundly

Frequent insufficient sleep and poor sleep patterns are chronic stressors. They increase the levels of stress hormones and pro-inflammatory cytokines. As a result, they not only reduce your fertility but impair your cognitive abilities and cause emotional problems.

During pregnancy, women who report more insomnia symptoms (such as difficulty in initiating and maintaining sleep, and early morning awakening) and/or poor sleep quality (do not feel refreshed after sleep) are more likely to have depressive symptoms. They are also more likely to develop postpartum depression. Besides, short sleep duration (< 7 hours per night) and/or poor sleep impair carbohydrate metabolism and increase the risk of gestational diabetes mellitus. Finally, short sleep duration (< 7 hours per night) is associated with longer labor duration and higher rates of cesarean births.

As insufficient sleep and poor sleep increase the level of stress hormones and pro-inflammatory cytokines and decrease the level of BDNF, they are detrimental to the developing fetus. Poor sleep quality during pregnancy has been associated with:

- A 1.25 times increased risk of preterm birth

Sleep lasting less than 8 hours per night has been associated with:

- A 3.80 times higher risk of miscarriage (spontaneous abortion) during the first and second trimester

- A 2.84 times higher risk of low birth weight

However, it has to be noted that the sleep duration here was based on maternal subjective report, and research suggests that pregnant women actually sleep 30 minutes less than they subjectively report.

Since people generally maintain the same sleep habits and sleep problems may persist for a while, it is important for women to establish healthy sleep patterns early on.

Sleep 8–9 hours per night

Although individual difference does exist, generally adults need 7–9 hour of sleep per day. However, as already noted, several studies suggest that, maternal sleep duration less than 8 hours per night is associated with poor birth outcomes. Oversleeping (sleep duration > 9 hours) is also detrimental to health, as it increases the risk of obesity. Therefore, 8–9 hours of sleep during pregnancy is preferable.

Tips to help you get better sleep

Obtaining enough sleep day-to-day obviously is highly important, but obtaining high-quality sleep is essential as well. You can take a sleep quality test at https://brainandlife.net/test-sleep-quality to check if you are sleeping well. A total score ≤ 5 indicates good sleep quality while a total score > 5 indicates poor sleep quality. If you score > 5, read the following tips carefully to ensure healthy sleep habits and refer to a doctor if necessary.

A dozen specific strategies that help optimize sleep are presented below:

- Establish more regularity and consistency in the timing of daily activities, especially the timing of getting up, evening meals, and bedtime routine. For example, you may want to read, take a hot shower, and then go to bed. Higher levels of regularity in behavioral rhythms are associated with better sleep outcomes, less depressive symptoms, and improved health.

- Make your bedroom quiet, cool, and dark, and your bed comfortable.

- Use your bedroom only for sleep, do not work or watch TV or videos in bed. This helps to establish a conditioning between your bedroom and sleep.

- Nap early, keep it short and before 5 p.m. Regular napping has been associated with enhanced mood, reduced risk of cardiovascular diseases and better cognitive functioning; but late napping may interfere with night sleep.

- Avoid caffeine, alcohol, and nicotine three to six hours prior to bedtime, as these chemicals interfere with sleep; not only this, avoid them at all costs because they are toxic to your baby.

- Avoid heavy meals 2–3 hours before bedtime. Eating big or spicy meals may cause discomfort and interfere with sleep. If you feel hungry, try a light snack at least 45 minutes before bedtime.

- Consume enough liquids during the day, so that you won't wake up thirsty nor have to go to bathroom in the middle of sleep.

- Do not use light-emitting electronic devices such as cell phones and tablets before bedtime, as it has negative effects on sleep.

- Exercise every day, as regular exercise improves sleep quality. But try to avoid vigorous exercise 2 hours before going to bed, for vigorous late-night exercise may produce increased arousal and prolong the time you take to fall asleep.

- Try to reduce total sitting time and time spent viewing television. The more total sitting time and time spent viewing television, the greater odds of taking a long time to fall asleep ($\geq$ 30 min), waking up too early in the morning and poor sleep quality, and the higher risk for obstructive sleep apnea (the most common sleep disorder that involves repeated pauses in breathing that occurs during sleep due to upper airway obstructions).

- If you can't fall asleep after 20–30 minutes, get out of bed, go to another room, and do something relaxing, for example reading or listening to slow, soothing music until you are tired enough to sleep.

- Don't stare at your clock at night. It actually increases stress and interferes with sleep.

CHAPTER 6
Stop Smoking

Smoking is one of the most harmful factors for health. There are over 4,000 chemicals in cigarette smoke including benzo(a)pyrene, nicotine, carbon monoxide and acrylamide, and many are carcinogens. Cigarette smoking, whether active or passive (second-hand smoke), substantially increases the risk of various cancers (such as lung cancer, oral cancer, laryngeal cancer, esophageal cancer, stomach cancer, cancer of the urinary bladder, pancreatic cancer, kidney cancer, cervical cancer, breast cancer, colorectal cancer, and liver cancer), cardiovascular diseases (coronary heart disease), respiratory diseases (COPD), dental diseases, cataract and macular degeneration, peptic ulcer disease, fractures, osteoporosis, and diabetes.

Smoking also reduces fertility and the quality of sperm and eggs. During pregnancy, smoking increases the risk of hypertension, preterm delivery, and the risk of stillbirth.

Many toxic chemicals cross the placenta and due to poor metabolism of the fetus, many of these chemicals turn out higher in concentration in the fetus than in the mother. For instance, it has been estimated that the fetal concentration of nicotine is 15% higher than that in the maternal body. These toxic chemicals directly damage the fetal brain and body and increase the risk of many fetal defects. Maternal smoking causes a twofold higher risk of atrial septal defects—a congenital heart defect with a hole in the wall that separates the top two chambers or atria of the heart.

The chemicals in cigarette smoke also have indirect detrimental effects on the fetus. Firstly, nicotine increases maternal blood pressure and heart rate and induces vasoconstriction of the uteroplacental vasculature, which reduces fetal blood circulation and in turn decreases the nutrients and oxygen available to the fetus. Secondly, nicotine suppresses maternal appetite, which causes poor nutrition of the mother and fetus. Thirdly, smoking causes severe inflammation in the maternal body and reduces her BDNF levels. Thus, offspring of mothers who smoked during pregnancy have:

- At fetal period: a smaller volume of the cerebellum and ventricular system

- At birth: a smaller volume of the cerebellum and frontal lobe

- At 10–13 years: a reduced gray matter (consisting of neuronal cell bodies) volume of the cerebral cortex

Consequently, children whose mothers smoked during pregnancy have poorer cognitive development:

- The Danish National Birth Cohort found that at 5 years of age, children of mothers who smoked >=10 cigarettes per day during pregnancy had 4 lower IQ points than those of non-smoking;

- The Swedish Cohort Study found that at 15 years of age, adolescents of mothers who smoked 1–9 cigarettes per day during pregnancy were 1.6 times more likely to perform poorly at school, whereas those of mothers who smoked >=10 cigarettes per day were 1.9 times more likely to perform poorly. (These findings do not suggest 9 cigarettes per day are equally as toxic as 1 cigarette per day and that 20 cigarettes per day are equally toxic as 10 cigarettes per day. We know that the more cigarettes smoked, the more dangerous.)

This reduced cognitive development and poor academic achievement has been confirmed in several large-scale studies conducted in the United States,

Canada, Australia, Spain, Taiwan, Poland, and South Korea. These studies further found that:

- The offspring of mothers who smoked during pregnancy exhibit various emotional and social problems: they are more impulsive, aggressive, more likely to experience negative emotions such as depression, at a higher risk of ADHD, and have more problems with their peers;

- The offspring of mothers who smoked during pregnancy are at a 1.5 times higher risk of being overweight;

- Smoking by the father or other household members at home when the mother does not smoke has similar detrimental effects on the development of the offspring.

Thus, cigarettes should be avoided altogether, not only in the pregnant mother but also in others household members.

Quitting abruptly works the best

Although most smokers prefer to quit gradually—to reduce the amount they smoke before quitting— rather than abruptly, it is nevertheless the latter that is more effective, as shown by a 2016 study conducted by Nicola Lindson-Hawley at the University of Oxford.

Lindson-Hawley and her colleagues looked at about 700 people who smoked at least 15 cigarettes a day, but were planning to quit on various quit dates. Half of them were randomly assigned to quit abruptly at their quit date, whereas the other half gradually reduced their smoking over the two weeks prior to their quit date. Both groups had behavioral support from nurses and used nicotine replacement before and after the quit day. As a result, it was found that at four weeks after the quit date, whereas 49% of the abrupt group were successful, 39% of the gradual-cessation group were successful; at six months after the quit date, whereas 22% of the abrupt group were successful, only 15.5% of the gradual-cessation group were successful. These results suggest that quitting smoking abruptly, or cold-turkey, is more likely to lead to lasting abstinence than quitting gradually.

It is recommended that you quit smoking as soon as possible; set a quit date, motivate yourself, tell your family, friends, and coworkers and ask them for support and understanding. You can read "A guide for tobacco users to quit"

(http://apps.who.int/iris/bitstream/10665/112833/1/978
9241506939_eng.pdf?ua=1)

and other resources developed by WHO
(http://www.who.int/tobacco/quitting/en/)

and U.S. Centers for Disease Control and Prevention
(https://www.cdc.gov/tobacco/data_statistics/fact_shee
ts/cessation/quitting/index.htm).

CHAPTER 7
Stop Drinking Alcohol

In a 2014 study, Philip A. May at the University of North Carolina at Chapel Hill set out to identify the most predictive maternal risks underlying offspring cognitive deficits at 6–7 years of age. He found that among a number of maternal characteristics, the late recognition of pregnancy and the quantity of alcoholic drinks consumed during the 3-month period before pregnancy, are the most predictive maternal risks. The quantity of drinks by the father was also predictive.

Parental alcohol drinking before conception induces germ line epigenetic changes that cause physiologic and behavioral abnormalities in their offspring. How does this toxic effect occur? Firstly, alcohol reduces the absorption of many nutrients especially vitamins like folate, thiamine, and B6. Secondly, alcohol inhibits the activity of IGF-1, which promotes growth in almost all the cells in the body, including sperm and oocytes. Thirdly, alcohol increases inflammation in the body. All these influences damage germ cells and induce germ line epigenetic modifications, which is inherited to the offspring.

In line with this, adoption studies have reported positive associations between reduced cognitive abilities in offspring and alcoholism in the biological but not the adoptive father. As new sperm are made every 42–76 days, damaged sperm can be replaced within 3 months of mitigated exposures. Therefore, fathers-to-be should stop drinking alcohol at least three months before planned pregnancy.

Alcohol consumption by the mother is far more catastrophic, as the fetus is harnessed in the mother's womb. In a 2015 study, Claire D. Coles at Emory University found that the more maternal peri-conceptual alcohol use, the poorer the mental development of the infant at 6 months of age. Whereas alcohol consumed before conception reduces fertility and causes germ line epigenetic modifications, alcohol consumed after conception causes direct damage to the fetus. As mentioned above, alcohol causes malnutrition, reduces the levels of growth factors, and induces inflammation. Furthermore, alcohol can cross the placenta and reach the fetal brain, where it induces abnormalities in glial cells, the latter provide nutrients to neurons. As a result, maternal consumption of alcohol reduces neuronal survival and causes severe damage to the fetal brain.

Fetal alcohol spectrum disorders (FASD) are a leading cause of developmental disabilities due to women's alcoholic habits prior to and during pregnancy. Affected infants not only show abnormal physical appearance, but also exhibit severely delayed cognitive and behavioral development. Actually, FASD perhaps is the single, most proven dangerous factor to the fetal brain. Affected infants have a smaller brain and a smaller volume in almost all the brain areas important for high-order cognitive, emotional and social processing, including the frontal, parietal, temporal, occipital cortex, the cerebellum, and the basal ganglia. Obviously, they show deficits in high-order functioning, possess lower IQ, report more memory and reasoning problems, are more likely to suffer from depression, anxiety, ADHD, addiction, and more likely to commit suicide, have poor communication and social skills and report a poor relationship with peers.

There is no known safe amount of alcohol use prior to or during pregnancy

All alcoholic beverages—including all wines, beer, and mixed drinks—can affect your baby's growth. In a study of almost 31,000 pregnancies, James L. Mills at the U.S. National Institute of Child Health and Human

Development set out to determine how much drinking by the mother during pregnancy is safe. Mills found that even less than one drink (e.g., half a drink) a day affects fetal growth and reduces birth weight. In a more recent study of over 9,000 children, Kapil Sayal at the University of Bristol, U.K. found that maternal consumption of even less than one drink per week during the first trimester causes significant mental health problems in the offspring at 4 and 7 years of age.

While writing this chapter, I heard people saying they or their pregnant family sometimes drank wine and cocktails during their last pregnancy and their baby turned out "fine." Similarly others say that their parents and parents' parents "weren't told any of this, and just went along with everything they did every day in their normal life, and a lot of those kids are quite normal." Still, others say that one glass of wine here or there is ok because "it calms the mother's mood which is better for the baby." These beliefs are very problematic. "Fine" and "normal" kids born to pregnant mothers who drank alcohols actually are not at their best potential. Damage has been done to the brain, even if that damage is not immediately noticeable. Some of the detrimental effects may not be realized until the children are in school, while some may not ever be known, because people seldom know what their children's best potential is, not to mention the fact that they often look at their children through rose-tinted glasses. Furthermore, one drink perhaps relaxes the mother, but the cost of this— the toxicity of alcohol — outweighs the small benefit. Besides, one always has many more effective, win-win strategies to manage one's stress and mood (see Chapter 11). The situation is the same for cigarettes smoking. Stay away from alcohol and cigarettes at all costs.

Here are several practical tips provided by The Drinkaware Trust, an independent UK alcohol education charity (https://www.drinkaware.co.uk/advice/how-to-reduce-your-drinking/how-to-cut-down/how-to-stop-drinking-alcohol-completely) as well as some support resources provided by the U.S. National Institute on Alcohol Abuse and Alcoholism (https://www.niaaa.nih.gov/alcohol-health/support-treatment).

CHAPTER 8
Maintain a Healthy Body Weight

Being either underweight or overweight are associated with lower fertility, in men and women. Underweight, namely a BMI of less than 18.5, suggests malnutrition and is associated with reduced levels of growth factors. Your BMI is calculated as your weight in kilograms divided by the square of your height in meters. Overweight, which is often divided into simply overweight ($25 \leq BMI < 30$) and obesity ($BMI \geq 30$), causes inflammation in the body, increases the level of the stress hormone cortisol and reduces the level of growth factors. Both underweight and overweight reduce the quality of sperm and eggs.

Much research has focused on the negative consequences of maternal underweight and overweight. For instance, maternal underweight has been associated with:

- Intrauterine growth restriction (which indicates a high developmental risk and is associated with cerebral palsy, cognitive deficits, behavioral problems, cardiovascular disease, type 2 diabetes, and stroke)

- A 1.24 times higher risk of spontaneous abortion

- A 1.29 times higher risk of preterm birth

- A 1.64 times higher risk of low birth weight

- Decreased language abilities at 12 months of age

- Delayed cognitive development at 24 months of age

Meanwhile, maternal obesity during pregnancy is associated with placental dysfunction and has been linked to:

- A 1.87 times higher risk of neural tube defect

- A 1.3 times higher risk of fetal death and miscarriage

- A 1.4–2 times higher risk of stillbirth

- An over 1.5 times higher risk of preterm birth

- A 1.2–1.4 times higher risk of low birth weight

- An over 2 times higher risk of large-for-gestational-age infants (indicating risks of obesity)

- A 1.38 times higher risk of neonatal intensive care use

- An over 3 times higher risk of childhood overweight/obesity

- 5 lower IQ points at 5 years of age

- More attention problems at school at 5 years of age

- A double higher risk of emotional problems at school at 5 years of age

- A 1.7 times higher risk of ADHD at 7 years of age

Therefore, adequate management of weight prior to conception is essential.

Underweight suggests malnutrition, or the consumption of energy and nutrients is not enough for the growing need of the body. On the other hand, overweight suggests an excessive intake of energy compared to energy expended. Overweight is also associated with nutritional deficiencies because of the poor nutritional quality of the food consumed; for instance, high saturated fat and sugar. So the management of weight is twofold, maintaining an adequate caloric intake and eating a balanced nutritious diet. For information on what composes a balanced nutritious diet, review Chapter 3. Here we will talk more about caloric intake.

The daily intake of calories

The daily intake of calories depends on gender, age, metabolism, and levels of physical activity. In general, people at 21–25 years of age who maintain a moderately active lifestyle (physical activity equivalent to walking for 30 minutes per day, in addition to the normal activities associated with independent living) need 2,800 kcal for men and 2,200 kcal for women per day. People at 26–45 years of age who maintain a moderately active lifestyle need 2,600 kcal for men and 2,000 kcal for women per day.

For starters, read food labels and pay attention to what and how much you eat now. You need to track your weight and set appropriate weight gain/loss goals if necessary.

Note that women have different weight gain goals before as compared to during pregnancy. In this chapter we are talking about weight management before pregnancy. For weight management during pregnancy, please read *The Seed of Intelligence: Boost Your Baby's Developing Brain through Optimal Nutrition and Healthy Lifestyle* or refer to the guidelines by the U.S. Institute of Medicine (https://www.nap.edu/catalog/12584/weight-gain-during-pregnancy-reexamining-the-guidelines).

Management of underweight

If you are underweight, before trying to put on weight, determine whether or not you are suffering from any medical conditions that have caused your underweight, for instance, an overactive thyroid gland or infections. Talk to your healthcare provider before making any major dietary changes.

If you are safe to put on weight, eat an additional one or two dishes with each meal, and/or eat more frequently—eat one or two healthy snacks between meals. For instance, you can try the following, which are estimated to contain roughly 200–300 kcal:

- Have an extra morning snack of fruit with yogurt and an extra serving of vegetables with supper

- Have an extra glass of milk with lunch and supper

- Have an extra afternoon or evening snack of whole grain cereal with milk and sliced fruit or chopped nuts

- Have an extra afternoon snack of half a sandwich or whole grain toast with nut butter and a small glass of 100% orange juice

- Have an extra afternoon snack of dry meat or fish and a small piece of bannock

Three points should be noted. First, although the goal is to gain weight and achieve a BMI between 18.5 and 25, a healthy diet is nevertheless the prerequisite, as an unhealthy diet high in saturated fat and sugar is detrimental to your health and the seeds of your baby's developing brain. Second, rather than abrupt weight gain, a gradual, steady weight gain is preferred. Third, although physical activity burns your energy and seems counterproductive to your goal of gaining weight, it is still highly recommended. Regular physical exercise enhances your immunity, reduces your risk of infection, and increases your levels of growth factors.

Management of overweight

Weight loss during pregnancy is not recommended as energy restriction is as detrimental to the fetus as obesity. Instead, obese women should lose 5–10% weight before conception.

As with being underweight, some medical conditions such as underactive thyroid and medications may cause you to gain weight. So it is recommended that you first talk to your healthcare provider and ask for a checkup. You can then make a weight loss plan with the help from your healthcare provider.

It's natural to want to lose weight very quickly. But evidence shows that people who lose weight gradually and steadily (about 0.5–1 kg per week) are more successful in maintaining that weight loss. Healthy weight loss usually takes 3–6 months (for losing 6–25 kg). Because weight loss isn't just about a "diet" or "program." It's about an ongoing lifestyle change in daily eating and exercise habits.

Overweight is the result of excessive caloric intake, especially from high saturated fat and high-carbohydrate foods. Exercise and dietary restriction are the two keys to losing excessive fat and keeping a healthy weight. Alone, both are effective at reducing weight, but it is the combination of them that achieves the biggest effect.

To lose weight, you must expend more calories than you take in. Likely, you will need to reduce your caloric intake by 500–1000 calories per day to lose about 0.5–1 kg per week. Actually, as demonstrated by dozens of well-controlled experiments, reducing caloric intake by 500–750 kcal/day effectively leads to weight loss in overweight and obese people.

For physical exercise, various scientific weight loss programs recommend at least 150 minutes of moderate-intensity exercise per week, and many people need more than 300 minutes of exercise per week. The latter is equal to at least 60 minutes a day, five days a week. You can do many different kinds of exercise that suit your preferences, such as brisk walking, running, jogging, swimming, sports, or resistance exercise.

Once you've achieved a healthy weight, by relying on healthy eating and physical exercise most days of the week, you are more likely to successfully keep the weight off for the long haul.

CHAPTER 9
Prevent Infections

Infection is the invasion of the body by microscopic organisms known as pathogens such as viruses, bacteria, and parasites. The body reacts to the infection by activating the immune system to control or eradicate these infectious pathogens. It also releases pro-inflammatory cytokines, which further activates the immune system to deal with the invasion.

In pregnant women, the most common viral infections include influenza and viral gastroenteritis, while the most common bacterial infections include respiratory infection (such as pneumonia), urinary tract infection, and genital infection including STDs. The most common parasites infection is malaria.

One thing we know about infections during pregnancy is that, compared to non-pregnant women, because of immunologic alternations, pregnant women are more severely affected by infections with some organisms, including influenza virus, hepatitis E virus (HEV), herpes simplex virus (HSV), and malaria parasites. For instance, during the 2009 flu pandemic, it has been estimated that pregnant women were up to 7.2 times more likely to be hospitalized for treatment, 7.4 times more likely to be admitted to an intensive care unit, and 10.2 times more likely to die than non-pregnant women. Similarly, pregnant women are 10 times more likely than other people to develop Listeria infection, an infection caused by Listeria monocytogenes often contained in high levels in raw sprouts and soft cheese made with unpasteurized milk.

Another thing to know is that infections during pregnancy not only severely affect the mother, but also the unborn baby. Severe infections induce a high degree of inflammation and may infect the placenta and fetus, which leads to miscarriage, stillbirth, preterm delivery, and intrauterine growth restriction. Mild infections that are not sufficient enough to induce labor, nevertheless, can induce intrauterine inflammation and damage fetal organs including the brain.

For instance, as shown in a structural magnetic resonance imaging experiment with rhesus monkeys conducted by Sarah J. Short at the University of North Carolina at Chapel Hill, maternal mild infection with influenza one month before term reduced gray matter (which includes the cell bodies of neurons) throughout the cortex (which is involved in every neural process) and while matter (which includes the synaptic connections between neurons) in the parietal cortex (which integrates sensory information) of the offspring at 1 years of age.

In other words, influenza causes long-lasting damage to the fetal brain, which in turn results in many cognitive and emotional problems. It has been estimated that:

- Maternal infection with influenza during pregnancy doubles the risk of infantile autism;

- Maternal infection with influenza in the first trimester (the first 12 weeks of pregnancy) increases the risk of offspring schizophrenia by 7-fold.

Maternal bacterial infection causes similar problems:

- Any maternal bacterial infection in the first trimester increases the risk of offspring schizophrenia by 2.5-fold;

- Any maternal bacterial infection in the second trimester (from week 13 to 27 of pregnancy) increases the risk of autism spectrum disorders by 1.4-fold.

Unfortunately, without special attention and preventive activities, a substantial proportion of women get infected during pregnancy. According to several large-scale surveys conducted in the United States and Europe, over half of pregnant women report taking at least one medication, whereas antibiotics are among the most commonly prescribed. Furthermore, it has been estimated that 11% of pregnant women get infected with influenza at some point, as high as 8% develop urinary tract infection, while 2% acquire genital herpes during pregnancy.

As we have already emphasized, the dilemma with infection (as with many other diseases) during pregnancy is that treatment is as detrimental to the fetus as the disease itself. Prevention is essential.

The primary way to prevent infection is to avoid exposure to infectious pathogens including viruses, bacteria, and parasites. Arm yourself with basic information about infectious diseases and avoid or reduce any potential exposure. Below are several helpful daily activities.

Follow good personal hygiene habits

Wash your hands well with soap and water well after the following:

- Using the bathroom

- Touching raw meat, raw eggs, or unwashed vegetables

- Preparing food and eating

- Gardening or touching dirt or soil

- Visiting or caring for a sick person

- Getting saliva (spit) on your hands

- Caring for and playing with children

- Changing diapers

- Before and after treating a cut or wound

- After touching an animal (including pet), animal feed, or animal waste

- After handling pet food or pet treats

- After touching garbage

Here is the handwashing method recommended by the U.S. Centers for Disease Control and Prevention:

- "Wet your hands with clean, running water (warm or cold), turn off the tap, and apply soap.

- Lather your hands by rubbing them together with the soap. Be sure to lather the backs of your hands, between your fingers, and under your nails.

- Scrub your hands for at least 20 seconds. Need a timer? Hum the "Happy Birthday" song from beginning to end twice.

- Rinse your hands well under clean, running water.

- Dry your hands using a clean towel or air dry them."

Pay attention to food safety

Many foods are contaminated by bacteria or parasites. As unpasteurized products are more likely to cause Listeria infection, avoid unpasteurized (raw) milk and foods (e.g., soft cheeses) made from it. Furthermore, cook foods thoroughly to kill bacteria and parasites. As an example, sprouts need warm and humid conditions to sprout and grow and unfortunately, these conditions are also ideal for the growth of bacteria, including Listeria, Salmonella, and E. coli. Do not eat raw or lightly cooked sprouts of any kind (including alfalfa, clover, radish, and mung bean sprouts). Cook sprouts thoroughly to kill the harmful bacteria.

For more information on food safety, visit https://www.foodsafety.gov held by U.S. Department of Health & Human Services.

Get vaccinated

Getting vaccinated is an essential part of staying healthy. Many serious infections can be prevented by immunization. While vaccines may cause some side effects, such as a temporarily sore arm or low fever, they are generally safe and effective.

Consult your healthcare provider regarding your immunization status and make sure your vaccinations are up to date. In general, women should get vaccinated for Hepatitis B and measles, mumps, and rubella (MMR) before pregnancy (in the case of MMR, at least 1–2 months before pregnancy, see Chapter 1). Furthermore, as recommended by the world health organization (WHO), influenza vaccination during any trimester is considered safe for both the mother and fetus, and all pregnant women can be vaccinated at any stage of pregnancy. It is equally important for the husband and other family members to get necessary vaccinations to reduce the risk of contagion.

Take travel precautions

If you are planning a trip, consult with your healthcare provider if you need any immunizations. Check the local information on infectious diseases before your trip and if possible, avoid visiting areas of ongoing infectious diseases such as dengue fever, yellow fever, and malaria.

Find more information on travel and health on the websites of WHO (http://www.who.int/topics/travel/en) and U.S. Centers for Disease Control and Prevention (https://wwwnc.cdc.gov/travel).

Prevent infections by sexual transmission

Engage in sexual relations only with one partner who has sex only with you. Both you and your partner should be tested for HIV and other STDs.

Boost your immune system

The secondary way to prevent infection is to boost your immune system, or build a strong body. Strategies introduced in the rest of the book are highly effective, including a nutritious diet, regular exercise, maintaining a healthy body weight (both being underweight and overweight are associated with reduced immunity and higher risk of infection), staying away from tobacco and alcohol, getting adequate sleep, building supportive social networks, and managing your stress and emotions.

CHAPTER 10
Promote Oral Health

We bring up the topic of oral health because of two reasons. First, dental disease is very common during pregnancy. It has been estimated that periodontal disease, including gingivitis (chronic infection of the gingiva or the superficial gum tissue) and periodontitis (chronic infection of the periodontium or the specialized tissues that both surround and support the teeth), affects nearly 100% pregnant women. Gingivitis is the most common oral disease and causes the gums to redden, swell, and bleed more easily. Periodontitis involves bacterial infiltration of the periodontium which produces toxins that stimulate a chronic inflammatory response. The periodontium is eventually broken down and destroyed, creating pockets.

Besides periodontal disease, dental caries is another condition that affects over 25% of women at reproductive age (people with periodontal disease are more likely to have dental caries). Dental caries is a disease in which dietary carbohydrate is fermented by oral bacteria into acid that demineralizes enamel.

Pregnant women are at higher risk of periodontal disease for several reasons. During pregnancy, dental inflammation is aggravated by fluctuations in hormone levels, which compromises normal immune response. Besides, the oral cavity is exposed more often to gastric acid due to frequent vomiting (occurs in early pregnancy) and acid reflux (occurs in late pregnancy), which erodes dental enamel. The elevated acidity and mucin levels in saliva further favor the formation of bacterial plaque, which eventually induces periodontal disease.

Of note, wisdom teeth or third molars, which appear at the back of the mouth in almost all adults, have a high chance of becoming a problem during pregnancy. Wisdom teeth commonly affect other teeth as they develop, becoming impacted (failing to emerge through the gums or emerge only partially) and causing pain, inflammation, and infection. Thus, wisdom teeth removal should be performed months before pregnancy to ensure optimal maternal health throughout pregnancy.

Maternal dental disease has been linked to pregnancy complications and negative fetal outcomes. It has been estimated that women who have periodontal disease during pregnancy have:

- An over double higher risk of preeclampsia

- An over 9-fold higher risk of gestational diabetes

- A 1.3 fold increased risk of stillbirth

- An almost 3-fold higher risk of preterm birth

A maternal oral screening test

In a 2016 study, Ajesh George at Western Sydney University developed a maternal oral screening test for antenatal clinic use. You can take this test here https://brainandlife.net/maternal-oral-screening-test to see whether you should get a dental check-up now.

Healthy diet for healthy teeth

In general, a balanced nutritious diet is essential for oral health. Several most important nutrients for oral health include vitamin A, C, D, calcium, and phosphorus. Vitamin A is important for the development of healthy bone and mucosa. Vitamin C prevents gum bleeding, promotes calcium absorption, and has anti-inflammatory effects. Vitamin D is important for bone development and the absorption and metabolism of calcium and phosphates. Calcium and phosphorus are important for bone development and teeth mineralization. Food resources of each nutrient are presented below:

- Vitamin A: orange-colored fruits and vegetables such as peaches, carrots, and red peppers

- Vitamin C: fruits and vegetables such as orange, lemon, grapefruit, kiwi, tomato, broccoli, and dark green leafy vegetables

- Vitamin D: dairy food, eggs, and seafood

- Calcium: dairy food, seafood, beans, dried fruits, broccoli, and dark green leafy vegetables

- Phosphorus: dairy, eggs, seafood, and meat

On the plus side, fresh fruits and vegetables that contain a high level of dietary fibers aid in cleaning teeth during chewing thus promoting good oral hygiene and reducing the risk of oral disease.

Oral hygiene

Here are several practical guidelines for oral hygiene.

- Brush at least twice daily;

- Brush with a soft toothbrush to lessen gum irritation;

- Floss at least once daily;

- Use periodic warm salt-water rinses to sooth tender gums;

- Refrain from consuming too much sugar and food that contains large amounts of sugar (e.g., candies, pastries), as they promote caries formation;

- Consume fruit juice, yogurt, and fermented milk with meals to reduce their cariogenic effects;

- After vomiting, rinse your mouth with baking soda mouthwash called sodium bicarbonate solution to neutralize acid and protect teeth.

CHAPTER 11
Enhance Mental Health

At no time more than now are we realizing the impact of mental health on our physical health, brain, and daily lives. Our mental health for instance in terms of the levels of stress can directly affect our physical health and our health behaviors, such as diet and exercise. Psychological stress, be it an argument, a failure at a job interview, financial constraints, or family conflicts, causes negative emotions and the release of stress hormones in the body. Long-lasting or repeated stress will induce a pro-inflammatory state in the body. Stress also reduces the levels of growth hormones. Consequently, damage to many organs occurs.

Furthermore, stress can directly affect our habits of health such as diet and exercise. The concepts of "emotional eating" and "comfort food" are not new. When stressed, people often eat junk foods, drink alcohol, or smoke to cope with the internal tension, which is actually unhealthy. The good news is there are two disciplines called psychosomatic medicine and health psychology that deal with these issues.

Equally important, chronic stress also impairs our productivity, work performance, and our ability to socialize. Workplace stress and executive burnout are hot topics in the study of industrial & organizational psychology.

Getting back to conception and pregnancy, like cigarettes and alcohol, stress reduces fertility in both men and women. As stress induces long-lasting changes in the body, maternal stress before and during pregnancy severely impacts the fetus. As one robust example, in a Danish national study of over 65,000 children, Jiong Li at the University of Aarhus, Denmark reported that children whose mothers were bereaved by death of a close family member within the period from a year before pregnancy until birth of the infants were at a 1.68 times higher risk of becoming overweight at 12 years of age. It suggests that even the maternal psychological state long before pregnancy has a far-reaching impact on the infant's development.

Infants born to stressed mothers exhibit broad developmental deficits in cognitive, emotional, behavioral, linguistic, motor skills, and in social functioning. They are also more susceptible to a wide range of psychopathology, including depression, autism, ADHD, conduct disorder, and schizophrenia. For instance, scientists have reported:

- At 8 months of age: lower mental development in infants whose mothers experienced high amounts of daily hassles in early pregnancy;

- Before 4 years old: delays in motor development and increased amounts of behavioral problems, including excessive clinging, crying, hyperactivity, low frustration threshold, and antisocial behavior in children whose mothers experienced severe and continuing familial or marital discord during pregnancy;

- At 6 years old: lower school scores of gymnastics, reading, writing, mathematics, music, and behavior in the first year of grammar school in children whose mothers experienced high levels of stress during pregnancy;

- At 7 years old: less focused attention in children whose mothers experienced more stressful life events during the first trimester (the first 12 weeks) of pregnancy;

- Before 20-32 years old: a 1.67 times higher risk of developing schizophrenia in the first 20-32 years of life in children whose mothers were exposed to death of a relative during the first trimester.

This evidence suggests that maternal mental health is important for a healthy pregnancy. Furthermore, psychological stress is contagious. Within a family, one person's stress and emotional state easily spill over to another. A couple's depressive symptoms are highly correlated, so the more depressed one person becomes, the more depressed the other grows. This is why stress management and mental health promotion is important for all family members.

You can check your levels of stress and negative emotions online here: https://brainandlife.net/psychological-tests/.

Most effective strategies

In a 2016 study, Maxime Taquet at Harvard Medical School set out to examine what people choose to do after experiencing negative emotions and what activities are the most effective in regulating emotions. Over a 4-week period, Taquet asked over 28,000 people to report their mood in real-time, and which activities they had been engaging in during that time via a smartphone application. Taquet found that, when people felt bad, they played sports most often. Following sports were spending time in nature, leisure activities, chatting with family or friends, and doing cultural activities.

Importantly, playing sports produced the most significant mood enhancement compared to the other activities. The ranking of the most effective strategies people used is shown here:

1. Sports

2. Spending time in nature

3. Cultural activities

4. Leisure activities

5. Chatting

Sports, as well as many other forms of physical exercise, greatly reduces stress and negative emotions. Going to parks, mountains, lakes, sea, and forest, engaging in various cultural (such as art, poetry, writing, photography, theatre, dance) and leisure activities (such as listening to music, reading, gardening) take one's attention away from the stressor, boosts positive emotions, and have been linked to better mental health. Chatting with family and friends gives people a sense of connection with others and this kind of social support exerts a robust stress coping effect (see next chapter). All of these strategies are more effective than drinking alcohol or eating. You can flexibly employ these effective strategies in your daily life.

It is time to enhance your emotional intelligence

Emotional wellbeing is not a personal thing; it is contagious. Therefore, managing your own as well as helping your partner and family members' emotions is a required for your baby's developing brain (and for your family harmony and wellbeing). Emotional intelligence involves the ability to identify, manage, and use your own and others' emotions. It consists of four areas:

- Accurately perceiving emotion: identifying emotions in facial expressions, voices, and body language;

- Understanding emotion: understanding that emotions are the expression of people's internal states;

- Using emotions to facilitate thought: using emotions as information or signals of people's internal states for thinking and reasoning;

- Managing emotion: effectively regulating emotions in oneself and others according to the situation.

People with high emotional intelligence have better familial and social relations, are perceived more positively by others, have higher life satisfaction, experience lower stress and depression, and possess better work performance and academic achievements.

Realizing the necessity of emotional intelligence is your first step towards better mental health and everyday living. As the next step, perhaps you can read Daniel Goleman's 1995 classic *Emotional Intelligence – Why It Can Matter More Than IQ* and my recent book *Psychology for Pregnancy: How Your Mental Health during Pregnancy Programs Your Baby's Developing Brain.*

CHAPTER 12
Achieve Family Harmony

Recent neuroscientific research has shown that viewing images of one's romantic partner activates almost the same neural reward circuitry as receiving monetary reward, viewing images of one's children, attractive faces, classic art, impressionist art, or landscapes, or listening to pleasurable music excerpts. Having a romantic partner is rewarding. Subsequently, reward induces positive emotions and reduces stress and negative emotions.

The importance of the romantic partner often is particularly appreciated in negative situations. When threatened by electric shock in the laboratory, compared to women holding a male stranger's hand or no hand at all, married women holding their husband's hand exhibited attenuated brain activation in areas representing threat responses such as the anterior insula. This threat buffering effect also varied as a function of marital quality so women with higher marital quality showed much less activation in the threat-related brain areas. Furthermore, while receiving painful thermal stimulation in the laboratory, women holding their romantic partner's hand or viewing their romantic partner's pictures reported less pain and exhibited reduced pain-related brain activation than those holding a stranger's hand or viewing pictures of a stranger.

Married people are healthier and happier

It is well-known in medical and psychological literature that married people on average are much healthier and happier than unmarried people. Among married people, those who report higher marital quality have better objective and subjective physical health, lower morbidity from cardiovascular disease, cancers, all-causes of mortality, faster wound healing, less pain-related disabilities, better sleep quality and cognitive function, greater life satisfaction and happiness, and lower depressive and anxiety symptoms. Higher marital quality also contributes to healthy behaviors, such as higher diet quality, less alcohol drinking, and greater adherence to medical recommendations.

Authentic partner support is a major source of high marital quality. When you perceive authentic support from your partner, you feel secure with him/her. You know your partner is always around when you are in need. You know he/she cares about your feelings and is a real source of comfort for you. You know you can share all your joys and sorrows with him/her.

Pregnant women with more partner support have fewer complications

The substantive evidence for the benefits of partner support underlines the profound role of the father for the pregnant mother (and vice versa). Pregnant women with more perceived support from their partners and who are more satisfied with their marriage show less pregnancy-related complications. They also report less stress, lower anxiety, and lower depression both during and following pregnancy. Their infants are more emotionally and cognitively competent, and less distressed in response to an unfamiliar place or stranger.

The cost of single-motherhood

In contrast, single-motherhood constitutes a risk for both the mother and fetus. Besides financial constraint, single mothers are more likely to experience emotional and behavioral issues. Single or new mothers not living with their partners report more or continued depressive symptoms during pregnancy and postpartum.

Furthermore, single mothers are more likely to have an unhealthy diet, consisting of:

- Lower intakes of fruits and vegetables

- Higher intake of high-fat foods

- Higher intake of sugar-sweetened beverages

- More frequent smoking habits

The reason for this unhealthy diet may include financial insecurity and feelings of stress and loneliness. As a result, single-motherhood is detrimental to fetal development. In a 2011 meta-analysis of 21 studies, Prakesh S. Shah at Mount Sinai Hospital estimated that compared to those born to married mothers, infants born to unmarried mothers have:

- A 1.46 times higher risk of low birth weight

- A 1.22 times higher risk of preterm birth

- A 1.45 times higher risk of small-for-gestational-age infants (indicating restricted fetal growth)

- An over double higher risk of childhood psychiatric disease

For single mothers, those living alone seem to be at a higher risk than those living with parents.

Given these findings, achieving family harmony and avoid single-motherhood is important.

The importance of family harmony

Family support, particularly from in-laws, is important for all expecting mothers. Family conflict is a potent stressor, while family support is a protective factor against almost all negative life events. Pregnant women who perceive more support from their family members report lower stress and less emotional problems both during and following pregnancy. They are less worried about their pregnancy and infants, less depressed, and less likely to get angry. They also show less pregnancy-related complications. Furthermore, their infants are more emotionally and cognitively competent.

Notably, here family harmony is the preferred term for family support, because family harmony is dynamic and involves support from and towards all other members. Pregnancy is not the work of the mother herself. Rather, it is a collaborative work among all the members. It is the role of all members of a family to create the most nourishing environment for the mother and fetus. This can be done a variety of ways, such as helping the mother to establish a nutritious diet, creating a cigarette smoke-free and psychological stress-free environment.

The other day I came across a young mother in an online pregnancy forum who just learned she was pregnant and was living with her boyfriend. She was in a dilemma: she wanted the baby, but her mother didn't like her boyfriend and didn't want them to marry. Worse, the young girl and her boyfriend did not have enough income to survive on their own and needed support from the girl's mother, and the boyfriend's parents were unavailable at that time due to unknown reasons. After our conversation, the young mother finally decided to move back in to live with her mother, receiving pregnancy care from her mother while trying her best to negotiate with her mother about her boyfriend so that they could get married and three of them could live together.

The growth of a baby in the womb is really fast and the surrounding physical and psychological environment of the mother, as you have seen throughout this book, exerts powerful, life-long impact on the baby. As such, it is essential for all family members to work together and construct the most nourishing environment for the mother and baby.

Good luck to the young mother, and good luck to you, dear reader.

CONCLUSION

Development psychologist Janet DiPietro at Johns Hopkins University once said, "Our old notion of nature influencing the fetus before birth and nurture after birth needs an update. There is an antenatal environment, too, that is provided by the mother." After the journey through this book, we know DiPietro's statement is very true, but still incomplete. The maternal antenatal environment during pregnancy is of critical importance; however, the nurture environment starts months long before conception, and is determined by both the mother and father.

There is no doubt that, for most people, bringing a new life into the world is the greatest joy they will experience, as well as one of the most challenging things they will face. However, as we have seen, conception and pregnancy is not the start. Rather, parents-to-be have to begin to prepare months before the planned conception. By making sure that your health is in top condition, you can safeguard your unborn child against a whole range of problems and give him the perfect start in life.

As the next step, I would recommend you read my series *"Your Baby's Developing Brain"* written for expecting parents, which gives you a more detailed account of how to achieve the most nourishing pregnancy.

To learn more about pregnancy and parenting and stay up to date with the latest research, please sign up for my newsletter at brainandlife.net and follow me on Twitter @ChongChenBlog.

Finally, if you enjoyed this book, please leave a brief review on Amazon or Goodreads to let more people discover it. Thanks.

REFERENCES

Preface

Finer, L. B., & Henshaw, S. K. (2006). Disparities in rates of unintended pregnancy in the United States, 1994 and 2001. *Perspectives on sexual and reproductive health*, *38*(2), 90-96.

Szwajcer, E., Hiddink, G. J., Maas, L., Koelen, M., & van Woerkum, C. (2012). Nutrition awareness before and throughout different trimesters in pregnancy: a quantitative study among Dutch women. *Family practice*, 29(suppl_1), i82-i88.

Goossens, J., Beeckman, D., Van Hecke, A., Delbaere, I., & Verhaeghe, S. (2017). PRECONCEPTION LIFESTYLE CHANGES IN WOMEN WITH PLANNED PREGNANCIES. *Midwifery*.

Chapter 1: Plan your pregnancy at least three months ahead

Frey, K. A., Navarro, S. M., Kotelchuck, M., & Lu, M. C. (2008). The clinical content of preconception care: preconception care for men. *American journal of obstetrics and gynecology*, *199*(6), S389-S395.

Sharma, R., Biedenharn, K. R., Fedor, J. M., & Agarwal, A. (2013). Lifestyle factors and reproductive health: taking control of your fertility. *Reproductive Biology and Endocrinology*, *11*(1), 66.

Coonrod, D. V., Jack, B. W., Boggess, K. A., Long, R., Conry, J. A., Cox, S. N., ... & Dunlop, A. L. (2008). The clinical content of preconception care: immunizations as part of preconception care. *American Journal of Obstetrics and Gynecology, 199*(6), S290-S295.

Atrash, H., Jack, B. W., Johnson, K., Coonrod, D. V., Moos, M. K., Stubblefield, P. G., ... & Reddy, U. M. (2008). Where is the "W"oman in MCH? *American Journal of Obstetrics and Gynecology, 199*(6), S259-S265.

Abbasi, J. (2017). The Paternal Epigenome Makes Its Mark. *Jama, 317*(20), 2049-2051.

Soubry, A., Hoyo, C., Jirtle, R. L., & Murphy, S. K. (2014). A paternal environmental legacy: evidence for epigenetic inheritance through the male germ line. *Bioessays, 36*(4), 359-371.

Cortessis, V. K., Thomas, D. C., Levine, A. J., Breton, C. V., Mack, T. M., Siegmund, K. D., ... & Laird, P. W. (2012). Environmental epigenetics: prospects for studying epigenetic mediation of exposure–response relationships. *Human genetics, 131*(10), 1565-1589.

Daxinger, L., & Whitelaw, E. (2012). Understanding transgenerational epigenetic inheritance via the gametes in mammals. *Nature reviews. Genetics, 13*(3), 153.

Skinner, M. K. (2014). Endocrine disruptor induction of epigenetic transgenerational inheritance of disease. *Molecular and cellular endocrinology, 398*(1), 4-12.

Huypens, P., Sass, S., Wu, M., Dyckhoff, D., Tschöp, M., Theis, F. ... & Beckers, J. (2016). Epigenetic germline inheritance of diet-induced obesity and insulin resistance. *Nature genetics*, *48*(5), 497-499.

Fontelles, C. C., Carney, E., Clarke, J., Nguyen, N. M., Yin, C., Jin, L. ... & De Assis, S. (2016). Paternal overweight is associated with increased breast cancer risk in daughters in a mouse model. *Scientific reports*, *6*, 28602.

Day, J., Savani, S., Krempley, B. D., Nguyen, M., & Kitlinska, J. B. (2016). Influence of paternal preconception exposures on their offspring: through epigenetics to phenotype. *American journal of stem cells*, *5*(1), 11.

Soubry, A., Schildkraut, J. M., Murtha, A., Wang, F., Huang, Z., Bernal, A. ... & Hoyo, C. (2013). Paternal obesity is associated with IGF2 hypomethylation in newborns: results from a Newborn Epigenetics Study (NEST) cohort. *BMC medicine*, *11*(1), 29.

Soubry, A., Murphy, S. K., Wang, F., Huang, Z., Vidal, A. C., Fuemmeler, B. F. ... & Hoyo, C. (2015). Newborns of obese parents have altered DNA methylation patterns at imprinted genes. *International journal of obesity (2005)*, *39*(4), 650.

Shnorhavorian M, Schwartz SM, Stansfeld B, Sadler-Riggleman I, Beck D, Skinner MK (2017) Differential DNA Methylation Regions in Adult Human Sperm following Adolescent Chemotherapy: Potential for Epigenetic Inheritance. *PLoS ONE* 12(2): e0170085.

Finegersh, A., Rompala, G. R., Martin, D. I., & Homanics, G. E. (2015). Drinking beyond a lifetime: New and emerging insights into paternal alcohol exposure on subsequent generations. *Alcohol*, *49*(5), 461-470.

Lambrot, R., Xu, C., Saint-Phar, S., Chountalos, G., Cohen, T., Paquet, M. ... & Kimmins, S. (2013). Low paternal dietary folate alters the mouse sperm epigenome and is associated with negative pregnancy outcomes. *Nature communications*, *4*, 2889.

McPherson, N. O., Bakos, H. W., Owens, J. A., Setchell, B. P., & Lane, M. (2013). Improving metabolic health in obese male mice via diet and exercise restores embryo development and fetal growth. *PloS one*, *8*(8), e71459.

Bielawski, D. M., Zaher, F. M., Svinarich, D. M., & Abel, E. L. (2002). Paternal alcohol exposure affects sperm cytosine methyltransferase messenger RNA levels. *Alcoholism: Clinical and Experimental Research*, *26*(3), 347-351.

Ashworth, C. J., Toma, L. M., & Hunter, M. G. (2009). Nutritional effects on oocyte and embryo development in mammals: implications for reproductive efficiency and environmental sustainability. *Philosophical Transactions of the Royal Society of London B: Biological Sciences*, *364*(1534), 3351-3361.

Hunt, P. A., & Hassold, T. J. (2008). Human female meiosis: what makes a good egg go bad? *Trends in Genetics*, *24*(2), 86-93.

Purcell, S. H., & Moley, K. H. (2011). The impact of obesity on egg quality. *Journal of assisted reproduction and genetics*, *28*(6), 517-524.

Velazquez, M. A., & Fleming, T. P. (2013). Maternal diet, oocyte nutrition and metabolism, and offspring health. In *Oogenesis* (pp. 329-351). Springer London.

Shaaker, M., Rahimipour, A., Nouri, M., Khanaki, K., Darabi, M., Farzadi, L. ... & Mehdizadeh, A. (2012). Fatty acid composition of human follicular fluid phospholipids and fertilization rate in assisted reproductive techniques. *Iranian biomedical journal, 16*(3), 162.

Hammiche, F., Vujkovic, M., Wijburg, W., de Vries, J. H., Macklon, N. S., Laven, J. S., & Steegers-Theunissen, R. P. (2011). Increased preconception omega-3 polyunsaturated fatty acid intake improves embryo morphology. *Fertility and sterility, 95*(5), 1820-1823.

Moran, L. J., Tsagareli, V., Noakes, M., & Norman, R. (2016). Altered preconception fatty acid intake is associated with improved pregnancy rates in overweight and obese women undertaking in vitro fertilisation. *Nutrients, 8*(1), 10.

Dunlop, A. L., Jack, B. W., Bottalico, J. N., Lu, M. C., James, A., Shellhaas, C. S., ... & Prasad, M. R. (2008). The clinical content of preconception care: women with chronic medical conditions. *American Journal of Obstetrics and Gynecology, 199*(6), S310-S327.

Uno, H., Eisele, S., Sakai, A., Shelton, S., Baker, E., DeJesus, O., & Holden, J. (1994). Neurotoxicity of glucocorticoids in the primate brain. *Hormones and behavior, 28*(4), 336-348.

Uno, H., Lohmiller, L., Thieme, C., Kemnitz, J. W., Engle, M. J., Roecker, E. B., & Farrell, P. M. (1990). Brain damage induced by prenatal exposure to dexamethasone in fetal rhesus macaques. I. Hippocampus. *Developmental Brain Research*, *53*(2), 157-167.

Moos, M. K., Dunlop, A. L., Jack, B. W., Nelson, L., Coonrod, D. V., Long, R. ... & Gardiner, P. M. (2008). Healthier women, healthier reproductive outcomes: recommendations for the routine care of all women of reproductive age. *American journal of obstetrics and gynecology*, *199*(6), S280-S289.

National Institute of Infectious Disease, Japan (2005). *Guidelines for Rubella vaccination*. Available at https://www.niid.go.jp/niid/images/idsc/disease/rubella/041119 /041119guide.pdf (last accessed 2017-11-18)

Chapter 2: Know the principle of parenting

This chapter is based on *The Seed of Intelligence*.

Chapter 3: Eat healthily

This chapter is based on *The Seed of Intelligence*.

Chapter 4: Be physically active

Nybacka, Å. Carlström, K., Ståhle, A., Nyrén, S., Hellström, P. M., & Hirschberg, A. L. (2011). Randomized comparison of the influence of dietary management and/or physical exercise on ovarian function and metabolic parameters in overweight women with polycystic ovary syndrome. *Fertility and sterility*, *96*(6), 1508-1513.

Rich-Edwards, J. W., Spiegelman, D., Garland, M., Hertzmark, E., Hunter, D. J., Colditz, G. A. ... & Manson, J. E. (2002). Physical activity, body mass index, and ovulatory disorder infertility. *Epidemiology*, *13*(2), 184-190.

Colberg, S. R., Sigal, R. J., Yardley, J. E., Riddell, M. C., Dunstan, D. W., Dempsey, P. C., ... & Tate, D. F. (2016). Physical activity/exercise and diabetes: a position statement of the American Diabetes Association. *Diabetes Care*, *39*(11), 2065-2079.

Gleeson, M., Bishop, N. C., Stensel, D. J., Lindley, M. R., Mastana, S. S., & Nimmo, M. A. (2011). The anti-inflammatory effects of exercise: mechanisms and implications for the prevention and treatment of disease. *Nature Reviews Immunology*, *11*(9), 607-615.

Chapter 5: Sleep soundly

This chapter is partly based on *The Seed of Intelligence*.

Kloss, J. D., Perlis, M. L., Zamzow, J. A., Culnan, E. J., & Gracia, C. R. (2015). Sleep, sleep disturbance, and fertility in women. *Sleep medicine reviews*, *22*, 78-87.

Chapter 6: Stop smoking

This chapter is partly based on *The Seed of Intelligence*.

Rom, O., Avezov, K., Aizenbud, D., & Reznick, A. Z. (2013). Cigarette smoking and inflammation revisited. *Respiratory physiology & neurobiology*, *187*(1), 5-10.

Bhang, S. Y., Choi, S. W., & Ahn, J. H. (2010). Changes in plasma brain-derived neurotrophic factor levels in smokers after smoking cessation. *Neuroscience letters*, *468*(1), 7-11.

Toledo-Rodriguez, M., Lotfipour, S., Leonard, G., Perron, M., Richer, L., Veillette, S. ... & Paus, T. (2010). Maternal smoking during pregnancy is associated with epigenetic modifications of the brain-derived neurotrophic factor-6 exon in adolescent offspring. *American Journal of Medical Genetics Part B: Neuropsychiatric Genetics*, *153*(7), 1350-1354.

Weng, S. F., Redsell, S. A., Swift, J. A., Yang, M., & Glazebrook, C. P. (2012). Systematic review and meta-analyses of risk factors for childhood overweight identifiable during infancy. *Archives of disease in childhood*, *97*(12), 1019-1026.

Kučienė, R., & Dulskienė, V. (2010). Parental cigarette smoking and the risk of congenital heart septal defects. *Medicina*, *46*(9), 635-641.

Lindson-Hawley, N., Banting, M., West, R., Michie, S., Shinkins, B., & Aveyard, P. (2016). Gradual versus Abrupt Smoking CessationA Randomized, Controlled Noninferiority TrialGradual Versus Abrupt Smoking Cessation. *Annals of internal medicine*, *164*(9), 585-592.

Chapter 7: Stop alcohol

This chapter is partly based on *The Seed of Intelligence*.

Hegedus, A. M., Tarter, R. E., Hill, S. Y., Jacob, T., & Winsten, N. E. (1984). Static ataxia: A possible marker for alcoholism. *Alcoholism: Clinical and Experimental Research*, 8(6), 580-582.

Tarter, R. E., Hegedus, A. M., Goldstein, G., Shelly, C., & Alterman, A. I. (1984). Adolescent sons of alcoholics: Neuropsychological and personality characteristics. *Alcoholism: Clinical and Experimental Research*, 8(2), 216-222.

Lieber, C. S. (2003). Relationships between nutrition, alcohol use, and liver disease. *Alcohol Research and Health*, 27, 220-231.

Van den Berg, H., van der Gaag, M., & Hendriks, H. (2002). Influence of lifestyle on vitamin bioavailability. *International journal for vitamin and nutrition research*, 72(1), 53-59.

González-Reimers, E., Santolaria-Fernández, F., Martín-González, M. C., Fernández-Rodríguez, C. M., & Quintero-Platt, G. (2014). Alcoholism: a systemic proinflammatory condition. *World Journal of Gastroenterology: WJG*, 20(40), 14660.

Coles, C. D., Kable, J. A., Keen, C. L., Jones, K. L., Wertelecki, W., Granovska, I. V. ... & Chambers, C. D. (2015). Dose and timing of prenatal alcohol exposure and maternal nutritional supplements: developmental effects on 6-month-old infants. *Maternal and child health journal*, 19(12), 2605.

May, P. A., Baete, A., Russo, J., Elliott, A. J., Blankenship, J., Kalberg, W. O. ... & Adam, M. P. (2014). Prevalence and characteristics of fetal alcohol spectrum disorders. *Pediatrics*, 134(5), 855-866.

Haycock, P. C. (2009). Fetal alcohol spectrum disorders: the epigenetic perspective. *Biology of reproduction, 81*(4), 607-617.

Resnicoff, M., Rubini, M., Baserga, R., & Rubin, R. (1994). Ethanol inhibits insulin-like growth factor-1-mediated signalling and proliferation of C6 rat glioblastoma cells. *Laboratory investigation; a journal of technical methods and pathology, 71*(5), 657-662.

Goodlett, C. R., & Horn, K. H. (2001). Mechanisms of alcohol-induced damage to the developing nervous system. *Alcohol research and health, 25*(3), 175-184.

Moore, E. M., Migliorini, R., Infante, M. A., & Riley, E. P. (2014). Fetal alcohol spectrum disorders: recent neuroimaging findings. *Current developmental disorders reports, 1*(3), 161-172.

Kodituwakku, P. W. (2009). Neurocognitive profile in children with fetal alcohol spectrum disorders. *Developmental disabilities research reviews, 15*(3), 218-224.

Mills, J. L., Graubard, B. I., Harley, E. E., Rhoads, G. G., & Berendes, H. W. (1984). Maternal alcohol consumption and birth weight: How much drinking during pregnancy is safe? *Jama, 252*(14), 1875-1879.

Crawford-Williams, F., Steen, M., Esterman, A., Fielder, A., & Mikocka-Walus, A. (2015). "My midwife said that having a glass of red wine was actually better for the baby": a focus group study of women and their partner's knowledge and experiences relating to alcohol consumption in pregnancy. *BMC pregnancy and childbirth, 15*(1), 79.

Chapter 8: Maintain a healthy body weight

This chapter is partly based on *The Seed of Intelligence.*

Ehrlich, S., Salbach-Andrae, H., Eckart, S., Merle, J. V., Burghardt, R., Pfeiffer, E. ... & Hellweg, R. (2009). Serum brain-derived neurotrophic factor and peripheral indicators of the serotonin system in underweight and weight-recovered adolescent girls and women with anorexia nervosa. *Journal of psychiatry & neuroscience: JPN, 34*(4), 323.

Caregaro, L., Favaro, A., Santonastaso, P., Alberinò, F., Di Pascoli, L., Nardi, M. ... & Gatta, A. (2001). Insulin-like growth factor 1 (IGF-1), a nutritional marker in patients with eating disorders. *Clinical Nutrition, 20*(3), 251-257.

Neggers, Y. H., Goldenberg, R. L., Ramey, S. L., & Cliver, S. P. (2003). Maternal prepregnancy body mass index and psychomotor development in children. *Acta obstetricia et gynecologica Scandinavica, 82*(3), 235-240.

US Department of Health and Human Services. (2015). 2015–2020 dietary guidelines for Americans. *Washington (DC): USDA.*

Johnston, B. C., Kanters, S., Bandayrel, K., Wu, P., Naji, F., Siemieniuk, R. A.... & Jansen, J. P. (2014). Comparison of weight loss among named diet programs in overweight and obese adults: a meta-analysis. *Jama,* 312(9), 923-933.

Miller, W. C., Koceja, D. M., & Hamilton, E. J. (1997). A meta-analysis of the past 25 years of weight loss research using diet, exercise or diet plus exercise intervention. *International journal of obesity*, 21(10), 941-947.

Chapter 9: Prevent infections

Kourtis, A. P., Read, J. S., & Jamieson, D. J. (2014). Pregnancy and infection. *New England Journal of Medicine*, *370*(23), 2211-2218.

Mosby, L. G., Rasmussen, S. A., & Jamieson, D. J. (2011). 2009 pandemic influenza A (H1N1) in pregnancy: a systematic review of the literature. *American journal of obstetrics and gynecology*, *205*(1), 10-18.

Goldenberg, R. L., Hauth, J. C. & Andrews, W. W. (2000) Mechanisms of disease: intrauterine infection and preterm delivery. *N. Engl. J. Med.* 342: 1500– 1507.

Giakoumelou, S., Wheelhouse, N., Cuschieri, K., Entrican, G., Howie, S. E., & Horne, A. W. (2015). The role of infection in miscarriage. *Human reproduction update*, 22(1), 116-133.

Elovitz, M. A., Brown, A. G., Breen, K., Anton, L., Maubert, M., & Burd, I. (2011). Intrauterine inflammation, insufficient to induce parturition, still evokes fetal and neonatal brain injury. *International Journal of Developmental Neuroscience*, 29(6), 663-671.

REFERENCES

Adams Waldorf KM, McAdams RM (2013) Influence of infection during pregnancy on fetal development. *Reproduction*. 146(5):R151-62

Desai, M., ter Kuile, F. O., Nosten, F., McGready, R., Asamoa, K., Brabin, B., & Newman, R. D. (2007). Epidemiology and burden of malaria in pregnancy. *The Lancet infectious diseases*, 7(2), 93-104.

Atladóttir, H. Ó., Thorsen, P., Østergaard, L., Schendel, D. E., Lemcke, S., Abdallah, M., & Parner, E. T. (2010). Maternal infection requiring hospitalization during pregnancy and autism spectrum disorders. *Journal of autism and developmental disorders*, 40(12), 1423-1430.

Short, S. J., Lubach, G. R., Karasin, A. I., Olsen, C. W., Styner, M., Knickmeyer, R. C., ... & Coe, C. L. (2010). Maternal influenza infection during pregnancy impacts postnatal brain development in the rhesus monkey. *Biological psychiatry*, 67(10), 965-973.

Brown, A. S., Begg, M. D., Gravenstein, S., Schaefer, C. A., Wyatt, R. J., Bresnahan, M. ... & Susser, E. S. (2004). Serologic evidence of prenatal influenza in the etiology of schizophrenia. *Archives of general psychiatry*, 61(8), 774-780.

Atladóttir, H. Ó., Henriksen, T. B., Schendel, D. E., & Parner, E. T. (2012). Autism after infection, febrile episodes, and antibiotic use during pregnancy: an exploratory study. *Pediatrics*, peds-2012.

Sørensen, H. J., Mortensen, E. L., Reinisch, J. M., & Mednick, S. A. (2008). Association between prenatal exposure to bacterial infection and risk of schizophrenia. *Schizophrenia bulletin*, *35*(3), 631-637.

Mitchell, A. A., Gilboa, S. M., Werler, M. M., Kelley, K. E., Louik, C., Hernández-Díaz, S., & Study, N. B. D. P. (2011). Medication use during pregnancy, with particular focus on prescription drugs: 1976-2008. *American journal of obstetrics and gynecology*, *205*(1), 51-e1.

Stephansson, O., Granath, F., Svensson, T., Haglund, B., Ekbom, A., & Kieler, H. (2011). Drug use during pregnancy in Sweden–assessed by the Prescribed Drug Register and the Medical Birth Register. *Clinical epidemiology*, *3*, 43.

Lupattelli, A., Spigset, O., Twigg, M. J., Zagorodnikova, K., Mårdby, A. C., Moretti, M. E. ... & Juraski, R. G. (2014). Medication use in pregnancy: a cross-sectional, multinational web-based study. *BMJ open*, *4*(2), e004365.

Andrade, S. E., Gurwitz, J. H., Davis, R. L., Chan, K. A., Finkelstein, J. A., Fortman, K., ... & Yood, M. U. (2004). Prescription drug use in pregnancy. *American journal of obstetrics and gynecology*, *191*(2), 398-407.

Irving, W. L., James, D. K., Stephenson, T., Laing, P., Jameson, C., Oxford, J. S. ... & Zambon, M. C. (2000). Influenza virus infection in the second and third trimesters of pregnancy: a clinical and seroepidemiological study. *BJOG: An International Journal of Obstetrics & Gynaecology*, *107*(10), 1282-1289.

Delzell JE Jr, Lefevre ML. (2000). Urinary tract infections during pregnancy. *Am Fam Physician*, *61*(3), 713-720.

Anzivino, E., Fioriti, D., Mischitelli, M., Bellizzi, A., Barucca, V., Chiarini, F., Pietropaolo, V. (2009). Herpes simplex virus infection in pregnancy and in neonate: status of art of epidemiology, diagnosis, therapy and prevention. *Virol J*. 6:40.

Beverly Merz (2016) *How to prevent infections: A few simple precautions can help you avoid getting sick with an infectious disease.* Available at https://www.health.harvard.edu/staying-healthy/how-to-prevent-infections (last accessed 2017-10-24)

Centers for Disease Control and Prevention (2017) *10 Tips for Preventing Infections Before and During Pregnancy.* Available at https://www.cdc.gov/pregnancy/infections.html (last accessed 2017-10-24)

WHO. (2012). Vaccines against influenza. WHO position paper–November 2012. *Wkly Epidemiol Rec*, *87*, 461-76.

Carroll, I. D., Toovey, S., & Van Gompel, A. (2007). Dengue fever and pregnancy—a review and comment. *Travel Medicine and Infectious Disease*, *5*(3), 183-188.

Jack, B. W., Atrash, H., Coonrod, D. V., Moos, M. K., O'donnell, J., & Johnson, K. (2008). The clinical content of preconception care: an overview and preparation of this supplement. *American journal of obstetrics and gynecology*, *199*(6), S266-S279.

Guerrant, R. L., Oriá, R. B., Moore, S. R., Oriá, M. O., & Lima, A. A. (2008). Malnutrition as an enteric infectious disease with long-term effects on child development. *Nutrition reviews*, *66*(9), 487-505.

Marti, A., Marcos, A., & Martinez, J. A. (2001). Obesity and immune function relationships. *Obesity reviews*, *2*(2), 131-140.

Chapter 10: Promote oral health

Silk, H., Douglass, A. B., Douglass, J. M., & Silk, L. (2008). Oral health during pregnancy. *American Family Physician*, *77*(8).

Minozzi, F., Chipaila, N., Unfer, V., & Minozzi, M. (2008). Odontostomatological approach to the pregnant patient. *Eur Rev Med Pharmacol Sci*, *12*(6), 397-409.

Russell, S. L., & Mayberry, L. J. (2008). Pregnancy and oral health: a review and recommendations to reduce gaps in practice and research. *MCN: The American Journal of Maternal/Child Nursing*, *33*(1), 32-37.

Pirie M et al (2007) Review dental manifestations of pregnancy. 9: 21-6

Merchant, A. T. (2012). Periodontitis and dental caries occur together. *The journal of evidence-based dental practice*, *12*(3 Suppl), 18-19.

Boggess, K. A., Lieff, S., Murtha, A. P., Moss, K., Beck, J., & Offenbacher, S. (2003). Maternal periodontal disease is associated with an increased risk for preeclampsia. *Obstetrics & Gynecology*, *101*(2), 227-231.

Xiong, X., Buekens, P., Vastardis, S., & Pridjian, G. (2006). Periodontal disease and gestational diabetes mellitus. *American journal of obstetrics and gynecology*, *195*(4), 1086-1089.

Mobeen, N., Jehan, I., Banday, N., Moore, J., McClure, E. M., Pasha, O. ... & Goldenberg, R. L. (2008). Periodontal disease and adverse birth outcomes: a study from Pakistan. *American journal of obstetrics and gynecology*, *198*(5), 514-e1.

Vergnes, J. N., & Sixou, M. (2007). Preterm low birth weight and maternal periodontal status: a meta-analysis. *American journal of obstetrics and gynecology*, *196*(2), 135-e1.

Wannamethee, S. G., Lowe, G. D., Rumley, A., Bruckdorfer, K. R., & Whincup, P. H. (2006). Associations of vitamin C status, fruit and vegetable intakes, and markers of inflammation and hemostasis. *The American journal of clinical nutrition*, *83*(3), 567-574.

Kloetzel, M. K., Huebner, C. E., & Milgrom, P. (2011). Referrals for dental care during pregnancy. *Journal of Midwifery & Women's Health*, *56*(2), 110-117.

Chapter 11: Enhance mental health

This chapter is partly based on *Psychology for Pregnancy*.

Sharma, R., Biedenharn, K. R., Fedor, J. M., & Agarwal, A. (2013). Lifestyle factors and reproductive health: taking control of your fertility. *Reproductive Biology and Endocrinology*, *11*(1), 66.

Li, J., Olsen, J., Vestergaard, M., Obel, C., Baker, J. L., & Sørensen, T. I. (2010). Prenatal stress exposure related to maternal bereavement and risk of childhood overweight. *PLoS One*, 5(7), e11896.

Chapter 12: Achieve family harmony

This chapter is partly based on *Psychology for Pregnancy*.

Shah, P. S., Zao, J., & Ali, S. (2011). Maternal marital status and birth outcomes: a systematic review and meta-analyses. *Maternal and child health journal*, *15*(7), 1097-1109.

Weitoft, G. R., Hjern, A., Haglund, B., & Rosén, M. (2003). Mortality, severe morbidity, and injury in children living with single parents in Sweden: a population-based study. *The Lancet*, *361*(9354), 289-295.

Crawford-Williams, F., Steen, M., Esterman, A., Fielder, A., & Mikocka-Walus, A. (2015). "My midwife said that having a glass of red wine was actually better for the baby": a focus group study of women and their partner's knowledge and experiences relating to alcohol consumption in pregnancy. *BMC pregnancy and childbirth*, *15*(1), 79.

INDEX

ABOUT THE AUTHOR

Chong Chen is a research scientist at the RIKEN Brain Science Institute in Wako, a suburb of Tokyo, Japan. He studied at Hokkaido University, where he obtained a Ph.D. in Medicine and won several academic awards, including the Takakuwa Eimatsu Award.

Chong has been the author of some 20 articles, all of which have been published in professional journals and which cover several aspects of his fields of expertise; neuroscience, psychiatry and psychology.

In addition to these important pieces, Chong has now written five books, including **Fitness Powered Brains: Optimize Your Productivity, Leadership and Performance**, which is ideal for business people, **Plato's Insight: How Physical Exercise Boosts Mental Excellence**, which shows how being physically active can directly correlate to mental ability and a series of three books called **Your Baby's Developing Brain**, which illustrates the recent scientific finding that babies' brains are developing long before they make their entrance into the world.

The three volumes focus on parental mental health, the optimal maternal nutrition and lifestyle and how the intelligent fetus learns and what parents can do to promote its learning.

When he has free time, Chong likes to get some fresh air and exercise by cycling. He also loves playing Ping-Pong, reads novels and poems and is a huge fan of the Argentine Tango.

As far as the future goes, Chong hopes that he will be able to translate scientific findings into ways that will allow regular people to live better lives. And through his books, he hopes that he can reach a much wider audience.

You can contact Chong Chen and follow what he is writing about at:

https://brainandlife.net
Twitter: @ChongChenBlog
Email: chen@brainandlife.net